RNA Viruses Infection

Edited by Yogendra Shah

Published in London, United Kingdom

RNA Viruses Infection
http://dx.doi.org/10.5772/intechopen.98167
Edited by Yogendra Shah

Assistant to the Editor: Jagadish Joshi

Contributors
Kelvin Melkizedeck Leshabari, Godfrey Chale, Rashid Salim, Oumerzouk Jawad, Klevor Raymond, Kissani Najib, Chraa Mohamed, Louhab Nissrine, Jayasri Das Sarma, Fareeha Saadi, Debanjana Chakravarty, Grishma Kasle, Masfique Mehedi, Sattya Narayan Talukdar, Babayemi Olawale Oladejo, Covenant Femi Femi Adeboboye, Rizaldy Taslim Pinzon, Chanda Siddoo-Atwal, Cristina Tudoran, Mariana Tudoran, Voichita Elena Lazureanu, Adelina Raluca Marinescu, Dorin Novacescu, Talida Georgiana Cut, Yogendra Shah, Jagadish Joshi

First published in London, United Kingdom, 2022 by IntechOpen
IntechOpen is the global imprint of INTECHOPEN LIMITED, registered in England and Wales, registration number: 11086078, 5 Princes Gate Court, London, SW7 2QJ, United Kingdom

British Library Cataloguing-in-Publication Data
A catalogue record for this book is available from the British Library

Additional hard and PDF copies can be obtained from orders@intechopen.com

RNA Viruses Infection
Edited by Yogendra Shah
p. cm.
Print ISBN 978-1-80355-666-6
Online ISBN 978-1-80355-667-3
eBook (PDF) ISBN 978-1-80355-668-0

Meet the editor

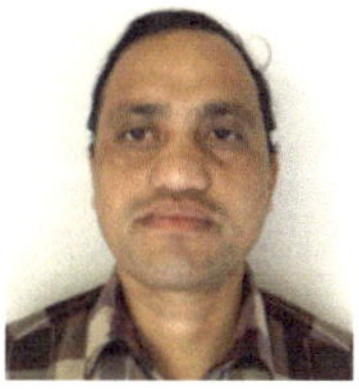

Dr. Yogendra Shah is a consultant microbiologist and lecturer at Seti Provincial Hospital COVID-19 PCR Lab and Kathmandu College of Science and Technology, Nepal. He completed his Ph.D. in Veterinary Medicine (Bacteriology) from the Graduate School of Veterinary Medicine, Hokkaido University, Japan in 2017. His research entails investigating the molecular epidemiological features/transmission dynamics of infectious diseases and zoonotic infectious diseases in Nepal using molecular techniques like ELISA, polymerase chain reaction (PCR), RT-PCR, loop-mediated isothermal amplification (LAMP), DNA sequencing, and whole genome sequencing (WGS). He was awarded the 2019 Young Science and Technology Award from the Nepal Academy of Science and Technology (NAST) and the 2021 Sudarpaschim Province Youth Scientist Award from the Province Youth Council. His research interests include infectious diseases, zoonotic infectious diseases, and vector-borne diseases. He has published more than forty-one research articles in peer-reviewed journals and twelve books.

Contents

Preface

RNA virus infections are a major health problem. There has been a sudden increase in cases of infectious diseases worldwide, including swine flu, MERS-CoV, and influenza virus SARS-COV2, which caused a devastating pandemic that killed millions of people. Since 1900, there have been ten pandemics, with viral orthomyxovirus and coronavirus being mostly responsible for eight. It might be genetic reassortment among human and animal viruses by the antigenic shift that results in new pandemic viruses; however, most research has revealed that origin is related to the zoonotic or interspecies transmission of viruses (e.g., coronavirus). Climate change also plays a significant role in the risk of arboviruses and rodent-borne viruses. To prevent future pandemics of RNA virus infections, constant surveillance in humans and animals as well as laboratory testing and screening, improved biosecurity measures, and more effective vaccines and broad-spectrum antivirals are needed.

This book examines pandemic-causing RNA viral infections, including SARS-CoV2, respiratory syncytial virus (RSV), influenza, HIV, and others. It provides information on molecular epidemiology features, transmission dynamics, pandemic outbreaks, pathogenesis, laboratory diagnosis, and prevention and control of RNA viruses using the One Health approach. Chapters address such topics as chronic inflammatory bowel disease and central nervous system demyelination, the role of IL6 in RNA virus infection, neurotropic virus-induced meningoencephalomyelitis, COVID-19 prevention through vitamins and supplements, aging and HIV risk in nonpregnant persons, RNA viruses in the tropics, and much more. Keywords: RNA virus, SARS-CoV2, Climate, Epidemiology, Diagnosis, Vaccine, One health.

Yogendra Shah
COVID-19 PCR Lab,
Seti Provincial Hospital,
Dhangadhi, Nepal

Section 1

Respiratory Syncytial Viruses (RSV)

Chapter 1

Introductory Chapter: Plan and Preparedness to Prevent and Combat against the Pandemic RNA Virus Infection

Yogendra Shah and Jagadish Joshi

1. Introduction

Emerging and re-emerging of infectious diseases are one of the major public health threats for human health population globally [1, 2]. Nonetheless, infectious disease remains huge burden in the least developing countries with low and lower-middle incomes [1]. Additionally, more deaths were records from emerging and re-emerging viral diseases and new virus infections in contrast to seasonal and endemic infection that continued throughout the twenty-first century [3]. For example, the world has been struggling with the epidemic of dengue virus, severe acute respiratory syndrome coronavirus 2 (SARS-CoV2), Middle East respiratory syndrome (MERS), Zika virus, influenza virus, rabies virus, Nipah virus, and Ebola virus as in **Table 1** [4].

Among infectious diseases, RNA viruses are one of the primary causes of human infection and the prognosis of wherever new RNA viruses are likely to be exposed is an important public health alarming like ongoing pandemic (SARS-CoV-2), and the causative agent of coronavirus disease 2019 (COVID-19) pandemic has been infected more than 5,20,373,492 million people with over 6,270,232 deaths globally as reported by WHO, May 14, 2022 [5]. For instance, COVID-19 pandemic had caused a huge devastating influence on lives and livelihoods around the worldwide [3]. Therefore, emerging and re-emerging infectious diseases remain as the significant causes of human and animal morbidity and mortality to significant health care expenses in developing as well as developed countries [1]. Mostly, human RNA virus can be evolved and discovery owing to socioeconomic, land use, climate, and biodiversity variables. Abnormally, vector-borne viruses and severely zoonotic viruses are more related to climate and biodiversity, whereas non-vector-borne viruses and human transmissible viruses are more connected with urbanization. According to previous studies, it is revealed that predicted areas are in three new regions including East and Southeast Asia, India, and Central America from 2010 to 2019, probably by increasing surveillance and diversity of their virome [6].

Monkey pox is caused by chicken pox virus, one of the viral zoonotic diseases that was first recognized in human in 1970 at Democratic Republic of the Congo in a 9-year-old boy and also has been reported since 1970 from 11 African countries. Monkey pox has been reported to be outbreak leading to more than 70 cases of

Years	Pandemics	Pathogens	Reservoir Host	Deaths (Mortality rate)	Reproduction number	Reference
1889–1893	Russian flu	Influenza A/H3N8?	Avian	1.5million (1.56%/1000)	2.15%	[10]
1918–1919	Spanish Flu	Influenza A/H2N2	Avian	50 million	2.4–10.6%	[10]
1957–1959	Asian Flu	Influenza A/H2N2	Avian	1.5–2 million (1.2–2.6%)	1.8%	[10]
1968–1970	Hong Kong Flu	Influenza A/H3N2	Avian	1 million (0.10–0.28%)	1.06–2.06%	[10]
2002–2003	Severe acute respiratory syndrome (SARS)	SARS-CoV1	Bats, palm civets	811 (9–10%)	2–4%	[10]
2009–2010	Swine Flu	Influenza A/H1N1	Pigs	18,209		[10]
2015-	Middle East respiratory syndrome (MERS)	MERS-CoV	Bats, dromedary camels	858 (30%)	048–8.59%	[10]
2019-ongoing	COVID-19	SARS-CoV2	Bats, pangolins, civet cat	7 million (0.6–2%)	1–2.56%	[10]

Table 1.
Pandemic of RNA viruses causing infection globally from 1983 to 2022.

monkey pox from US (September 2018), UK (September 2018; December 2019; May 2021; and May 2022), Singapore (May 2018), and USA (July–November 2021). According to promedmail.org, recently have been identified the confirmed cases of monkey pox virus from Spain (14 cases; May 2022), France (1 cases; May 20, 2022), Belgium (2 cases), Germany (1 case), Italy (1 case; May 19, 2022), Sweden (1 case, May 19, 2022), Portugal (14 cases), UK (9 cases, May 6, 2022), Canada (2 cases), and Australia (1 cases, May 20, 2022) with cases fatality ratio around 3–6% [7, 8]. Additionally, WHO have been also reported the virus named called as acute hepatitis of unknown origin as April 21, 2022 with at least 169 cases from 11 countries located in the WHO European Region and one country in the WHO Region of the Americas (**Table 1**) [9].

One health approach should be rigorously engaged to detect new RNA virus cases, by surveillance as well as isolated and separate the suspected human and animal, laboratory diagnosis of infectious and zoonotic diseases, and treating them by providing early warning to veterinary and human public health authorities [10–13]. This chapter will provide the overview essence on globally concern and emerging public health RNA virus infections such as SARS-CoV2, RSV, Influenza virus, HIV, and others. The main importance of this chapter was to clearly understand the molecular epidemiology pattern, transmission dynamics, host response, viral evolution, molecular biology, pathogenesis mechanism of viral infection, diagnosis, and control about the RNA virus infection. This study will be help to provide the updating research information to the policy maker or planner for further diagnosis and treatment with genotyping tools, control, and prevention for further outbreak of diseases from RNA viruses' infection in tropical and subtropical countries by employing the One Health approach.

Author details

Yogendra Shah[1*†] and Jagadish Joshi[2†]

1 Seti Provincial Hospital, Dhangadhi, Kailali, Nepal

2 Health Directorate, Rajpur, Dipayal, Doti, Nepal

*Address all correspondence to: yogendra90@hotmail.com

† Equally contribution.

References

[1] Mourya DT et al. Emerging/re-emerging viral diseases and new viruses on the indiam horizon. The Indian Journal of Medical Research. 2019;**149**:447-467

[2] Tong S, Ebi K, Olsen J. Infectious disease, the climate and the future. Environmental Epidemiology. 2021;**5**:e133

[3] Baker RE et al. Infectious disease in an era of global change. Nature reviews. 2022;**20**:193-205

[4] Brown A, Horton R. A planetary health perspective on COVID-19: A call for papers. Lancet. 2020;**395**:1099

[5] World Health Organization (WHO). Health Emergency Dashboard. Available from: https://covid19.who.int/

[6] Zhang F et al. Global discovery of human-infective RNA viruses: A modelling analysis. PLoS Pathogens. 2020;**16**(11):e1009079

[7] Available from: https://www.who.int/news-room/fact-sheets/detail/monkeypox

[8] Available from: https://promedmail.org/

[9] Available from: who.int/emergencies/disease-outbreak-news/item/2022-DON376

[10] WHO. Nipah virus outbreaks in the WHO South-East Asia Region. Available from: http://www.searo.who.int/entity/emerging_diseases/links/nipah_virus_outbreaks_sear/en/. [Accessed: June 22, 2018]

[11] Shah Y, Paudel S, Pandey K, Gupta GP, et al. Insights into transmission dynamics of Mycobacterium tuberculosis complex in Nepal. Tropical Medicine and Health. 2022;**50**(1):8

[12] Chattu VK, Kumar R, Kumary S, Kajal F, David JK. Nipah virus epidemic in southern India and emphasizing "one health" approach to ensure global health security. Journal of Family Medicine and Primary Care. 2018;**7**:275-283

[13] Piret J, Boivin G. Pandemics throughout history. Frontiers in Microbiology. 2021;**11**:631736

Chapter 2

Respiratory Syncytial Virus

Sattya Narayan Talukdar and Masfique Mehedi

Abstract

Respiratory Syncytial Virus (RSV)-driven bronchiolitis is one of the most common causes of pediatric hospitalization. Every year, we face 33.1 million episodes of RSV-driven lower respiratory tract infection without any available vaccine or cost-effective therapeutics since the discovery of RSV eighty years before. RSV is an enveloped RNA virus belonging to the *pneumoviridae* family of viruses. This chapter aims to elucidate the structure and functions of the RSV genome and proteins and the mechanism of RSV infection in host cells from entry to budding, which will provide current insight into the RSV-host relationship. In addition, this book chapter summarizes the recent research outcomes regarding the structure of RSV and the functions of all viral proteins along with the RSV life cycle and cell-to-cell spread.

Keywords: RSV, RNA virus, RNA genome, replicative cycle, fusion protein, cell-to-cell spread, filopodia

1. Introduction

Human respiratory syncytial virus (RSV), despite being a human virus, was first isolated in 1955 from a chimpanzee with respiratory illness [1]. Since its first discovery, it did not take long to isolate RSV from infants with respiratory diseases. Indeed, serological studies verified the existence of RSV infection in infants and children [2, 3]. Now, RSV infection is a prominent cause of lower respiratory tract diseases (bronchiolitis and pneumonia) and hospitalization in children worldwide [4]. According to the most recent virus taxonomy, RSV now belongs to a new family *Pneumoviridae* of the order *Mononegavirales* [5].

2. RSV virion

RSV is an enveloped and cytoplasmic virus with non-segmented, negative-sense, single-stranded RNA genome [6]. RSV virions are known to bud out on the infected cell surface. The filamentous virion is up to 12 μm in length and 60 to 200 nm in diameter (**Figure 1**) [7–9]. RSV virions can be irregular-shaped spherical particles with a diameter ranging from 100 to 350 nm. Both filamentous and spherical virus particles mostly remain cell-associated [9].

IntechOpen

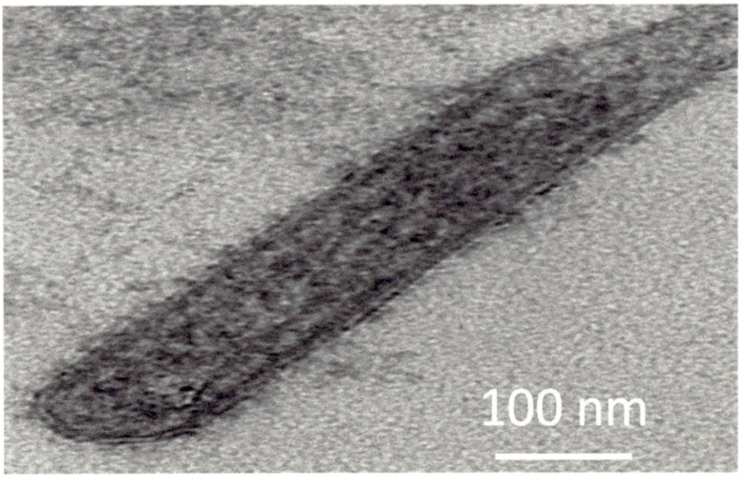

Figure 1.
RSV virion. A photomicrograph of an RSV filamentous virion. The image was taken under electron microscope.

3. RSV strains

There are two RSV strains as RSV A and RSV B and are categorized on basis of genetic and antigenic differences [10]. However, mostly extensive antigenic and nucleotide sequence variation was observed between RSV A and RSV B, however, genetic as well as antigenic variability was also studied within the individual groups of RSV [11]. Multiple studies demonstrated the differences in viral replication between these two groups; specifically, RSV A replicated to higher titers than RSV B viruses in both cell culture and animal models [12–16]. In addition, RSV A infection is more virulent and severe than RSV B [17].

4. RSV RNA and proteins

The RSV genome is a single-stranded, negative-sense RNA whose length is ranging from 15,191 to 15,226 nucleotides [9]. The RSV genome contains ten genes in the order 3′-NS1-NS2-N-P-M-SH-G-F-M2-L-5′ that are transcribed sequentially into 10 independent messenger RNAs (mRNAs) (**Figure 2**). Each RSV mRNA encodes a single major protein except for M2, which encodes two separate open reading frames (ORF) for M2–1 and M2–2 proteins, respectively [9, 18–20]. The M2–1 and M2–2 ORF are located in the upstream and downstream parts of the mRNA, respectively [9]. Like many RNA viruses, RSV brings ribonucleoprotein (RNP) complex as a piece of transcriptional machinery for its genome transcription and replication inside the infected cell cytoplasm. The RNP complex consists of the viral genome, nucleoprotein (N), phosphoprotein (P), and RNA-dependent RNA polymerase [L) [21].

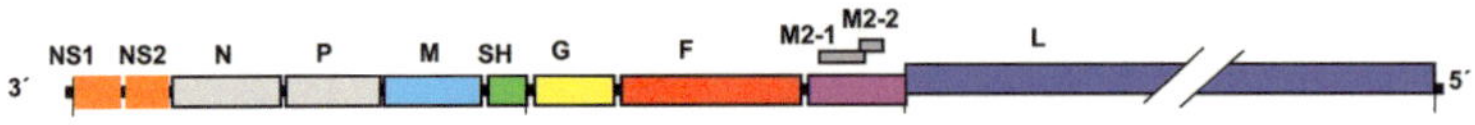

Figure 2.
Schematic of an RSV genome. RSV genome is a negative-sense non-segmented single-stranded RNA. The genome contained 10 genes oriented from 3′ end: NS1, NS2, N, P, M, SH, G, F, M2 (M2–1 and M2–2), and L.

4.1 Nucleoprotein (N)

The RNA genome is wrapped by N (391 amino acids) to create a nuclease-resistant, helical RNP complex called nucleocapsid (NC), and it functions as the template for both replication and transcription [22, 23]. RSV virus genome for replication does not follow the "rule of six" [24], which is common to most paramyxoviruses [25]. The three-dimensional (3D) crystal structure revealed a decameric, ribonucleoprotein complex of N protein and RNA with 3.3 A° resolution and suggested N protein can function as a helicase to separate temporary double-stranded RNA during RNA synthesis [23]. As a decameric structure, every N subunit has a core region comprising two domains, N-terminal and C-terminal, which are linked by a hinge region and the RNA genome turns inside a basic surface groove located at the interface of N-terminal/C-terminal; specifically, every N subunit interacts with seven ribonucleotides of RNA [23].

4.2 RNA-dependent RNA polymerase (L)

The L protein (2165 amino acids) has three enzymatic domains including RNA-dependent RNA polymerase (RdRp) domain, polyribonucleotidyl transferase domain which is essential for capping located in its N-terminal, and methyltransferase domain which is necessary for cap methylation located in C-terminal [26–29]. Viral mRNA undergoes a post-transcriptional modification before translation and methyltransferase plays a significant role by catalyzing the methylation of cap structure at both N7- and 2′-O-positions because N7-methylation is vital for viral RNA translation and 2′-O-methylation is important for hiding viral RNA from the innate immunity system [30].

4.3 Phosphoprotein (P)

The P protein (241 amino acids) is a homotetrameric protein consisting of N-terminal domain, oligomerization domain, and C-terminal domain and it functions as a cofactor of RdRp and plays a significant role in transcription and replication by networking with other RSV proteins [31–35]. P protein functions as a multimodular adaptor for RNA synthesis by interacting with N-RNA, L, and M2–1 [36]. P can act as a chaperone for newly synthesized N (N^0) protein by forming an N^0-P complex that prevents the association of N^0 with host RNA [37]. This protein is heavily phosphorylated by host kinase enzymes and it has 41 serine and threonine residues as potential phosphorylation sites; specifically, phosphorylation at residues T105, T188, T210, and S203 are essential for replication, and phosphorylation at residue S156 is vital for viral RNA synthesis [38].

4.4 RSV glycoproteins

As an enveloped virus, the RSV lipid envelope contains three transmembrane glycoproteins including a fusion (F) protein, an attachment glycoprotein (G), and a small hydrophobic (SH) protein; F and G proteins are essential for viral attachment and entry whereas SH protein is less likely involved in viral entry and budding [39, 40].

4.4.1 Fusion (F) protein

Fusion protein is a type 1 transmembrane protein (574 amino acids including a cytoplasmic tail domain of approximately 24 residues) involved in viral entry and assembly [39, 41]. Initially, F protein is synthesized as F0 protein and subsequently, F0 undergoes post-translational modification with multiple N-linked glycosylations depending on RSV strains [42]. To obtain fusion competence, precursor F0 protein (approximately 68–75 KDa) undergoes proteolytic cleavage by furin-like protease which cleaves two polybasic sites and removes a glycosylated peptide of 27 amino acids (Peptide 27 or Pep27) [43, 44]. This cleavage process occurs in the trans-Golgi network and then fusion protein transport to plasma membrane generating two subunits: one is amino-terminal F2 subunit (approximately 15–20 KDa) and another is carboxy-terminal F1 subunit (approximately 50–55 KDa) [45, 46]. A heterodimeric protomer is formed by F1 and F2 subunits covalently connected by disulfide bonds and three protomers combinedly form the matured trimeric form of F protein [47]. After trimerization, F protein exists as a prefusion conformation remaining approximately 12 nm above the membrane of the virus [48]. This prefusion conformation is not a stable form and undergoes a refolding process [6, 49]. This refolding process creates a more stable post-fusion conformation of F protein remaining approximately 17 nm above the viral membrane [50, 51]. The sequence difference of F ectodomains is almost 5% between RSV A and RSV B and therefore, F protein undergoes less antigenic drift and gets preference for suitable vaccine candidates [52].

4.4.2 Attachment glycoprotein (G)

In RSV-infected cells, G protein can exist in two forms; one is a membrane-bound form responsible for viral attachment and another is a secreted isoform responsible for immune evasion [53, 54]. The membrane-bound form (298 amino acids) is a type 2 integral membrane protein [55]. G protein has an amino-terminal cytoplasmic domain and a hydrophobic transmembrane domain; moreover, its ectodomain which undergoes post-translational modification with 4–5 N-linked glycans and 30–40 O-linked glycans, has two mucin-like regions and heparin-binding domains [55–57]. The translation of secreted G protein starts at an alternative AUG (Met48) located in the transmembrane domain allowing the ectodomain to secrete from the cell [58]. Both membrane-bound and secreted forms of G proteins are thought to be involved in RSV pathogenesis [59]. The higher variation of the mucin-like domain caused two subtypes of RSV: RSV A and RSV B [60].

4.4.3 Small hydrophobic (SH) protein

SH glycoprotein is a small transmembrane protein (64 amino acids for RSV A and 65 amino acids for RSV B) attached by a hydrophobic signal-anchor sequence closer to the N-terminal with extracellular C-terminal orientation; in addition, this protein is considered as less immunogenic because of smaller size and lower abundance during RSV infection [61]. It can exist in several forms including full-length form or post-translational modified form by glycosylation and phosphorylation [62]. Although its function is not clearly understood like other glycoproteins, several studies suggested SH protein can play an auxiliary role during viral fusion along with F glycoprotein; however, SH protein is not crucial for viral entry and syncytium formation [63–65]. SH protein primarily amasses in the lipid raft membrane of the Golgi complex and endoplasmic reticulum; however, lower levels of SH protein are associated with the envelope of filamentous virus [40]. SH protein did not play an essential role during viral replication in cell culture but SH-deleted RSV infection caused 10-fold lower titers in animal models [39, 66]. It can induce membrane permeability and form pentameric ion channels suggesting its role as viroporins which are short (approximately 100 amino acids) membrane proteins forming oligomers to act as ion channels [67]. Moreover, SH protein is essential to activate the NLRP3 inflammasome [68, 69]. The role of SH protein on apoptosis is not clear because RSV infected A549 cells produced TNF-α and cells were not sensitive to TNF-α-induced death but cells demonstrated a higher level of apoptosis after SH-deleted RSV infection indicating that RSV SH protein may affect the TNF-α pathway resulting in apoptosis delay by an alternative mechanism [70].

4.5 RSV matrix proteins (M and M2)

RSV has two matrix proteins including M protein and M2 protein [58].

4.5.1 M protein

M protein (256 amino acids) is a non-glycosylated protein located in the innermost part of the viral envelope [71]. It is the main protein responsible for viral assembly and budding by interacting with the cell membrane, viral envelope, and viral nucleocapsid [72, 73]. M protein has a zinc finger domain, two clusters of basic amino acids indicating a nuclear localization signal and two nuclear export signals and its N-terminal has lower hydrophobicity; in contrast, C-terminal has higher hydrophobicity [74]. M protein contains multiple phosphorylation sites and undergoes phosphorylation during infection but it is unclear whether these phosphorylations control its function [75]. During the early phase of infection, M protein is present in the host nucleus and inhibits host cellular transcription [76]. During the late phase of infection, M protein is mostly cytoplasmic, interacts with nucleocapsid, and inhibits the activity of viral transcriptase [77]. M protein is located in the cytoplasmic part of the plasma membrane-associated with the lipid rafts along with G and N proteins implying that lipid rafts can function as a platform for the assembly and budding of RSV [73]. M protein is active in a dimer form and the conversion of M-M dimer to oligomer is essential for viral assembly because the interference of dimer formation reduces viral filament maturation and budding [21].

4.5.2 M2 (M2-1 and M2-2) protein

M2–1 and M2–2 are nucleocapsid associated proteins [78]. RSV M2 gene has two overlapping ORFs as M2–1 and M2–2 [79]. The recent crystal structure of the M2–1 (194 amino acids) protein has revealed its native tetrameric form with 2.5 Å resolution and each of its monomers contains three domains including zinc-binding, oligomerization, and core domains [80, 81]. M2–1 functions as a transcriptional anti-terminator and processivity factor [79, 82]. M2–1 did not affect genome and antigenome synthesis indicating that M2–1 is not involved in RNA replication [79, 83]. M2–2 protein (90 amino acids) acts as a regulatory factor switching from transcription to RNA replication because mRNA accumulation was intensely higher after 12–15 hours of infection and then flattened in case of wild-type virus infection but M2–2 knockout virus infection showed continued accumulation [80]. Another study showed M2–2 protein could negatively regulate transcription and positively modulate RNA replication because recombinant RSV infection without NS1 and M2–2 protein demonstrated ten times lower viral growth kinetics in the upper respiratory tract of infants [84].

4.6 RSV nonstructural (NS) proteins (NS1 and NS2)

RSV NS proteins including NS1 (139 amino acids) and NS2 (124 amino acids) play a crucial role in interfering with host innate immunity by forming a "Nonstructural degradosome complex" which can act as a proteasome-like complex that disintegrates a massive number of proteins involved in the innate immune system [85, 86]. Infection with NS1 and NS2 single- and double-gene-deleted RSV demonstrated that both proteins function individually and jointly to accomplish the complete inhibitory effect on type I and III IFNs whereas NS1 has a more individual function [87, 88]. Both NS1 and NS2 target retinoic acid-inducible gene I (RIG-I) like receptors (RLRs), which are considered as host pattern recognition receptors for RIG-I and melanoma differentiation-associated gene 5 (MDA5) [89]. Both NS1 and NS2 induce multiple chemokines and cytokines like RANTES, IL-8, TNFα during viral infection [90]. RIG-I activation by ubiquitination is vital for stimulating antiviral response and tripartite motif-containing protein 25 (TRIM25)-mediated K63-polyubiquitination is essential for RIG-I activation [91]. NS1 protein inhibits RIG-I ubiquitination by interacting with TRIM25 and eventually suppresses type-I interferon (IFN) signaling [92]. Cytosolic NS1 can go to the host nucleus and interacts with the gene regulatory domains of immune response genes, which can control gene transcription and eventually modulates host response against RSV infection [93]. NS1 localized to mitochondria inhibits type-I interferon (IFN) signaling by binding with mitochondrial antiviral signaling protein (MAVS) because the MAVS-RIG-1 complex is essential for type-I IFN activation [94]. NS1 also stimulates miR-29a expression, which affects mRNA coding for interferon alpha/beta receptor 1 (IFNAR1) [95]. NS1 enhances autophagy by the mTOR pathway, which is beneficial for RSV replication but inhibits apoptosis and multiple inflammatory cytokines and IFN-α [96]. Recombinant RSV (NS-deficient) infection showed that mostly NS1 (partially NS2) inhibits the maturation of Dendritic cells, which in turn activates B and T cell responses [97]. NS1 can also inhibit the anti-inflammatory effect of glucocorticoids [98]. The recent X-ray crystal structure of NS2 reveals that it has a unique fold that allows to target molecules different from NS1 and activates distinct IFN antagonism pathway compared to NS1 [99]. Recombinant RSV virus without NS2 showed lower viral growth indicating the role of NS2 in viral replication by evading host immunity [100]. The increased level of IFNβ was not as high when recombinant RSV without NS1 or NS1/NS2 were applied suggesting that both NS1 and NS2 work together for interferon signaling suppression [84]. NS2 also plays a significant role in NF-κB activation, which can initiate a cascade by binding transcription promoters of several proinflammatory cytokines along with IRF-3 and IFN-α/β [90]. In addition to innate immunity, NS2 interferes with adaptive immunity by suppressing CD8+ T-cell responses as a consequence of controlling type 1 IFN [101]. Mostly NS2 along with NS1 play a role in delaying apoptosis, which can enable prolonged RSV replication by activating 3-phophoinositide-dependent protein kinase (PDK)-RAC serine/threonine-protein kinase-glycogen synthase kinase (GSK) pathway [102]. In addition, NS2 plays a significant role in modulating cell morphology, which causes the shedding of infected cells and the spreading of RSV virions [103].

5. Replicative cycle of RSV

5.1 Entry

RSV infection mostly occurs in the apical side of ciliated cells and type 1 pneumocyte; however, several reports suggested the presence of RSV RNA in the extrapulmonary sites and fluids, but more investigations are required [104–107]. RSV entry has two major phases; the first step is virion attachment to the host cell and the next step is the fusion of viral and host cell membranes in which host factors can involve in both or any individual phases [52]. Heparin-binding domain located between mucin-rich domains of G protein interacts with the unbranched disaccharide polymers specifically glycosaminoglycans (GAGs) connected to transmembrane proteins on the cell surface for the attachment observed in multiple cell culture studies [108–110]. Variation of G protein lacking heparin-binding domain showed viral attachment indicating the involvement of other regions of G protein during attachment [108]. Negatively charged regions of heparin sulfate contribute mostly and iduronic acid-containing GAG contributes minimally to the attachment [111–113]. Heparan sulfate proteoglycans (HSGP) act as the receptor for G protein in cell lines; however, recombinant RSV without G protein showed its infectivity; in contrast, HSGP does not express in ciliated epithelial cells, but G protein is still essential for infection in vivo [114–116]. However, the apical side of ciliated cells, which is the major site of RSV infection lack heparin sulfate indicating the involvement of other host factors, specifically, fractalkine receptor CX3C-chemokine receptor 1 (CX3CR1) bind to CX3C motif of G protein for the attachment [117, 118]. CX3CR1 expressed on the ciliated cells, acts as the receptor of G protein by interacting with its CX3C motif and mutations in the CX3C motif of G protein reduces RSV infection in vivo [117, 119–121]. F protein is involved in the viral attachment because RSV lacking G and SH proteins grows in cell culture studies and it interacts with heparin sulfate like G protein causing attachment and subsequent infection [63, 122, 123]. Almost 50% infection was observed after heparinase treatment and without GAG synthesis while RSV has F protein suggesting the interaction of F with other host factors; particularly, F protein facilitates entry by interacting with intercellular adhesion molecule 1, insulin-like growth factor 1, epidermal growth factor receptor, and nucleolin [124–127]. Host and viral membrane then fuse after attachment so that viral particles can enter the cytoplasm and this fusion process is p^H-independent and insensitive to lysosomal acidification [128, 129]. RSV infection induces an actin mediated rearrangement followed by plasma membrane blebbing and excess fluid uptake causing internalization of viral particles in a Rab5 positive macropinisome and this endocytic entry depends on the activation of F protein by a second proteolytic cleavage catalyzed by furin-like enzymes after endocytosis observed in A549 cell [130].

5.2 Transcription and replication

RSV replication and transcription are dependent on viral components including viral RNA, N, P, L, and M2–1 [131]. RSV utilizes its own machinery (RNP complex) to replicate in the host cytoplasm [132]. Inclusion body formation is a hallmark of RSV infection produced by multiple viral proteins including N, P, L, and M2–1 and this cytoplasmic structure is increased with RSV infection in epithelial cells [72, 133, 134]. Specifically, N and P proteins are important for inclusion body formation because the expression of these proteins with or without RSV infection showed inclusion body formation [135]. P protein can hijack host cell machinery by forming a complex with host phosphatase (PP1) and this P-PP1 complex dephosphorylates M2–1, as a result, P protein can recruit M2–1 protein in the inclusion body to facilitate viral RNA synthesis [136]. M protein is also reported to localize in inclusion bodies mediated by M2–1 protein [137]. The inclusion body is thought to be the first place where M protein interacts with the ribonucleoprotein complex and M protein is involved in the release of RNP from inclusion bodies towards budding [138]. Host actin cytoskeleton and Hsp70 proteins are also observed in inclusion bodies, but their role is not clear yet and they perhaps facilitate viral machinery [139]. RSV infection causes vigorous stress on the host cell resulting formation of cytoplasmic stress granules, which are different from cytoplasmic inclusion bodies and these stress granule formations facilitates viral replication [140].

Both viral RNA replication and mRNA transcription start from the same single promoter in leader (le) region (44-nucleotide long) at the 3′ end of RSV genome and it produces methyl-guanosine capped and polyadenylated mRNA during transcription and antigenome during replication [20, 141–143]. Each RSV gene has two conserved cis-acting elements including a gene start (gs) signal at the beginning and a gene end (ge) signal at the end [144]. The promoter of leader (Le) region at the 3′ end of RSV genome has two initiation sites, one is at position +1 or 1 U required for replication and another one is at position +3 or 3C required for transcription [145]. 9 out of 10 gs signaling sequences are highly conserved whereas the tenth one has minimal sequence difference in RSV genome [19]. During transcription, both gs and ge signaling sequences play significant role, specifically, gs signal provides direction to RNA-dependent RNA-polymerase (RdRp) for initiating RNA synthesis and ge signal provides direction to RdRp to polyadenylate and release the mRNA [146, 147]. Then RdRp connected to the template can initiate transcription again at the next gs signal and this process persists along RSV genome [144]. During replication, RdRp attaches a similar promoter sequence in le region, but it ignores ge signal and continues to proceed throughout the genome to produce an antigenome, which is a full-length positive-sense complement of RSV genome [145]. Viral genome and antigenome RNA are encapsidated in RSV nucleoprotein whereas viral mRNAs are not encapsidated [145]. Every nucleoprotein monomer interacts with 7 nucleotides of viral RNA and this complex forms a helical nucleocapsid acting as a template for the next RNA synthesis. This encapsidation is thought to increase RdRp activities to override ge signal during replication, therefore, encapsidation is the distinguishing factor between replication and transcription [23, 148, 149]. The trailer (tr) region (155-neucleotide long) at the 3′ end of RSV antigenome has a promoter, which allows RdRp towards RSV genome synthesis [142, 143, 150]. The first 12 nucleotides of tr promoter are like those of the le promoter and the signal starts from position +1 and + 3 undergoes replication and transcription, respectively, but tr promoter cannot produce capped and polyadenylated mRNA because of lacking ge signal sequence adjacent to tr promoter [151, 152]. However, it is reported that tr promoter can initiate transcription of short RNA, which can inhibit cellular stress granules [153]. The concentration of ATP or GTP can determine the fate of replication and transcription at positions +1 (1 U) or position +3 (3C) observed at in vitro model, specifically, higher ATP concentration stimulates initiation from 1 U and evades initiation at 3C, in contrast, higher GTP concentration displays opposite effect [154]. Overall, L and P proteins form the core RdRp and L-P complex then form L-P-N and L-P-M2–1 complex to initiate replication and transcription, respectively [79, 155].

5.3 Virion assembly and budding

Both assembly and budding of RSV occur at the apical side of ciliated cells [156]. RSV assembly is associated with lipid microdomain or lipid raft rich in cholesterol and sphingolipids; specifically, RSV filament formation observed in caveolin-1 and lipid-raft ganglioside GM1 rich regions of host cell surface membrane [157–159].

RSV assembly into viral filament occurs at the cell surface requiring the activity of F protein cytoplasmic tail and M protein and this process are not dependent on actin polymerization [160]. However, Mehedi et al., showed the depletion of ARP2 resulted in perturbation of RSV progeny virion on the infected cell surface, consequently reducing viral shedding [8]. Viral assembly requires the activity of F protein cytoplasmic tail and M protein because both proteins accumulate in inclusion bodies cytoplasmic tail of F protein enables the release of the complex of matrix and RNP from inclusion bodies [161]. Although previous studies showed that three proteins including M, P, and F proteins are enough to create virus-like particles, a recent nuclear magnetic resonance study suggests that three novel interaction sites of M on P including site I in α_{N2} region, site II in 115 to 125 region and oligomerization domain where oligomerization domain is necessary for virus-like structure formation and virus release [137]. The incorporation of RSV proteins into lipid microdomains during virus assembly can cause the interaction of F protein with host factors including caveolin-1, CD44, RhoA, causing microvillus-like projections essential for virus filament and syncytium formation [162, 163]. Actin cytoskeleton and actin-associated pathways linked with PI3K and Rac GTPase are involved in RSV assembly [164]. M protein can bind DNA as well as RNA and it localizes into the nucleus mediated by importin-β1 nuclear import receptor, which forms a complex with guanine nucleotide-binding protein Ran and binds M protein amino acid 100–183 [165, 166]. During the early phase of infection, nuclear accumulation of M protein was observed when M protein interacts with nuclear components mediated by its zinc finger domain resulting in the inhibition of host cell transcription [165]. During the later phase of infection, M protein undergoes phosphorylation inducing nuclear export mediated by Crm1 by unmasking the nuclear export signal [78]. Therefore, M protein is thought to play a regulatory role as a transcription inhibitory factor by inhibiting viral transcriptase to facilitate RSV assembly and budding [77, 167]. RSV glycoprotein and RNP vesicles combined together prior to the filamentous virus formation and G protein recycling has been observed via clathrin-mediated endocytosis, which might be connected with filamentous RSV formation [168]. RSV budding preferentially appears at the apical membrane of epithelial cells by an apical recycling endosome (ARE)-mediated apical protein sorting pathway [169]. RSV budding is independent of the endosomal sorting complex necessary for transport (ESCRT) mechanism controlled by ARE-associated protein, Rab11 family interacting protein 2 (FIP2) [170]. Recently, ARP2 is identified as a novel host factor of RSV budding and cell-to-cell spread [8].

6. RSV cell-to-cell spread

Although RSV progeny virions mostly remain cell-associated, virus shedding occurs from the infected cell's surface and through cellular protrusions namely filopodia [8, 9]. RSV-induced syncytium (multinucleated cell) formation is a common feature of RSV infection in vitro. The syncytium involves the merging of infected cells with the adjacent uninfected cells, which allows the transfer of viral components from infected cells to the adjacent uninfected cells [171] (**Figure 3**). Mehedi et al., first showed that RSV uses a novel filopodia-driven cell-to-cell spread mechanism in the lung epithelial cells in vitro (**Figure 4**). It appears that RSV infection modulates cellular actin dynamics; particularly, actin-related protein 2/3 (ARP2/3) complex-driven actin polymerization contributes to lamellipodium and filopodium formation

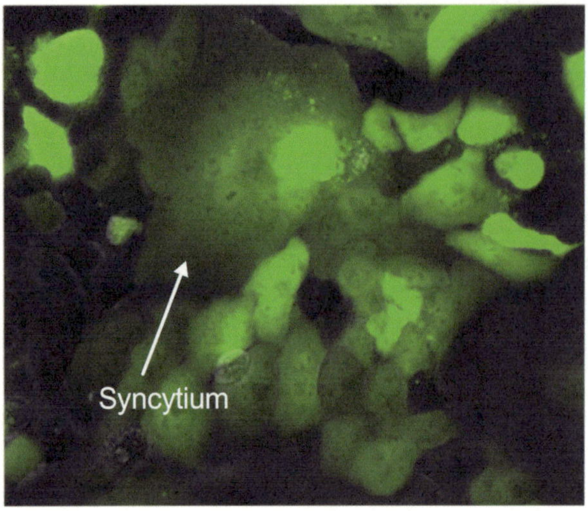

Figure 3.
RSV-induced syncytium (multinucleated cell) formation. A549 cells were infected with GFP-expressing RSV (RSV-GFP) at a multiplicity of infection of 1. At 48-hour post-infection, cells were fixed and imaged under an epifluorescence.

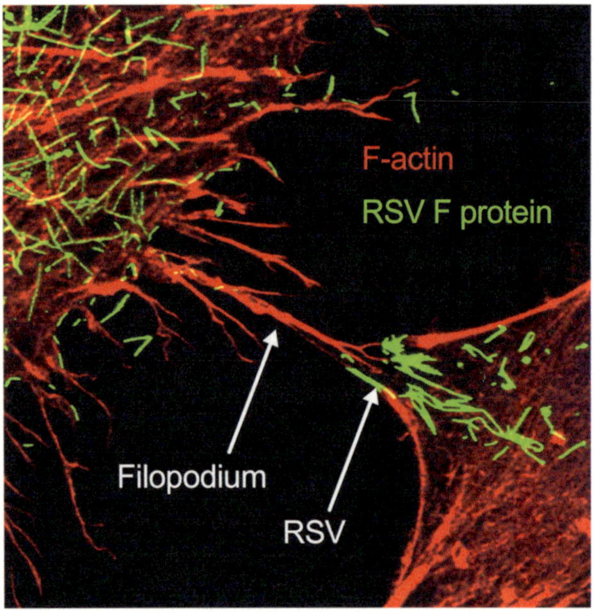

Figure 4.
Filopodia-driven RSV cell-to-cell spread. A549 cells were infected with RSV-WT (strain A) at a multiplicity of infection of 1. At 24-hour post-infection, cells were fixed, permeabilized, and stained for RSV F protein by using F-specific immunofluorescence (IFA) (green). F-actin was detected by rhodamine phalloidin staining (red). The image was taken under a stimulated emission depletion (STED) microscope.

of cell motility. They showed the depletion of ARP2, a major constituent of the ARP2/3 complex resulted in a substantial reduction of RSV budding and filopodia-driven cell-to-cell spread [8, 172–174].

Author details

Sattya Narayan Talukdar and Masfique Mehedi*
School of Medicine and Health Sciences, University of North Dakota,
Grand Forks, ND, USA

*Address all correspondence to: masfique.mehedi@und.edu

References

[1] Morris J, Blount R Jr, Savage R. Recovery of cytopathogenic agent from chimpanzees with goryza. Proceedings of the Society for Experimental Biology and Medicine. 1956;**92**(3):544-549

[2] Moris JABR, Savage RE. Recovery of cytopathic agent from chimpanzees with coryza. Proc Sci Exp Biol Med. 1956;**92**:544-550

[3] Chanock R, Finberg L. Recovery from infants with respiratory illness of a virus related to chimpanzee coryza agent (CCA). II. Epidemiologic aspects of infection in infants and young children. American Journal of Hygiene. 1957;**66**(3):291-300

[4] Verwey C, Nunes MC. RSV lower respiratory tract infection and lung health in the first 2 years of life. The Lancet Global Health. 2020;**8**(10):e1247-e12e8

[5] Rima B, Collins P, Easton A, Fouchier R, Kurath G, Lamb RA, et al. ICTV virus taxonomy profile: Pneumoviridae. Journal of General Virology. 2017;**98**(12):2912-2913

[6] Liljeroos L, Krzyzaniak MA, Helenius A, Butcher SJ. Architecture of respiratory syncytial virus revealed by electron cryotomography. Proceedings of the National Academy of Sciences. 2013;**110**(27):11133-11138

[7] Ke Z, Dillard RS, Chirkova T, Leon F, Stobart CC, Hampton CM, et al. The morphology and assembly of respiratory syncytial virus revealed by cryo-electron tomography. Viruses. 2018;**10**(8):446

[8] Mehedi M, McCarty T, Martin SE, Le Nouen C, Buehler E, Chen YC, et al. Actin-related protein 2 (ARP2) and virus-induced Filopodia facilitate human respiratory syncytial virus spread. PLoS Pathogens. 2016;**12**(12):e1006062

[9] Collins PL, Karron RA. Respiratory syncytial virus and Metapneumovirus. In: Knipe DMH, PM editor. Fields Virology. Sixth ed. Philadelphia: Lippincott Williums & Wilkins; 2013

[10] Mufson MA, Örvell C, Rafnar B, Norrby E. Two distinct subtypes of human respiratory syncytial virus. Journal of General Virology. 1985;**66**(10):2111-2124

[11] Storch GA, Park CS. Monoclonal antibodies demonstrate heterogeneity in the G glycoprotein of prototype strains and clinical isolates of respiratory syncytial virus. Journal of Medical Virology. 1987;**22**(4):345-356

[12] Crowe JE Jr, Bui PT, Firestone C-Y, Connors M, Elkins WR, Chanock RM, et al. Live subgroup B respiratory syncytial virus vaccines that are attenuated, genetically stable, and immunogenic in rodents and nonhuman primates. Journal of Infectious Diseases. 1996;**173**(4):829-839

[13] Hierholzer J, Tannock G, Hierholzer CM, Coombs R, Kennett ML, Phillips P, et al. Subgrouping of respiratory syncytial virus strains from Australia and Papua New Guinea by biological and antigenic characteristics. Archives of Virology. 1994;**136**(1-2):133-147

[14] Morgan L, Routledge E, Willcocks M, Samson A, Scott R, Toms G. Strain variation of respiratory syncytial virus. Journal of General Virology. 1987;**68**(11):2781-2788

[15] Stott E, Taylor G, Ball L, Anderson K, Young K, King A, et al. Immune and histopathological responses in animals vaccinated with recombinant vaccinia viruses that express individual genes of human respiratory syncytial virus. Journal of Virology. 1987;**61**(12):3855-3861

[16] Sullender WM, Anderson K, Wertz GW. The respiratory syncytial virus subgroup B attachment glycoprotein: Analysis of sequence, expression from a recombinant vector, and evaluation as an immunogen against homologous and heterologous subgroup virus challenge. Virology. 1990;**178**(1):195-203

[17] Walsh EE, McConnochie KM, Long CE, Hall CB. Severity of respiratory syncytial virus infection is related to virus strain. Journal of Infectious Diseases. 1997;**175**(4):814-820

[18] Collins PL, Wertz GW. cDNA cloning and transcriptional mapping of nine polyadenylylated RNAs encoded by the genome of human respiratory syncytial virus. Proceedings of the National Academy of Sciences. 1983;**80**(11):3208-3212

[19] Collins PL, Dickens LE, Buckler-White A, Olmsted RA, Spriggs MK, Camargo E, et al. Nucleotide sequences for the gene junctions of human respiratory syncytial virus reveal distinctive features of intergenic structure and gene order. Proceedings of the National Academy of Sciences. 1986;**83**(13):4594-4598

[20] Dickens L, Collins P, Wertz G. Transcriptional mapping of human respiratory syncytial virus. Journal of Virology. 1984;**52**(2):364-369

[21] Förster A, Maertens GN, Farrell PJ, Bajorek M. Dimerization of matrix protein is required for budding of respiratory syncytial virus. Journal of Virology. 2015;**89**(8):4624-4635

[22] Bhella D, Ralph A, Yeo RP. Conformational flexibility in recombinant measles virus nucleocapsids visualised by cryo-negative stain electron microscopy and real-space helical reconstruction. Journal of Molecular Biology. 2004;**340**(2):319-331

[23] Tawar RG, Duquerroy S, Vonrhein C, Varela PF, Damier-Piolle L, Castagné N, et al. Crystal structure of a nucleocapsid-like nucleoprotein-RNA complex of respiratory syncytial virus. Science. 2009;**326**(5957):1279-1283

[24] Samal SK, Collins PL. RNA replication by a respiratory syncytial virus RNA analog does not obey the rule of six and retains a nonviral trinucleotide extension at the leader end. Journal of Virology. 1996;**70**(8):5075-5082

[25] Kolakofsky D, Pelet T, Garcin D, Hausmann S, Curran J, Roux L. Paramyxovirus RNA synthesis and the requirement for hexamer genome length: The rule of six revisited. Journal of Virology. 1998;**72**(2):891-899

[26] Clarke MO, Mackman R, Byun D, Hui H, Barauskas O, Birkus G, et al. Discovery of β-d-2′-deoxy-2′-α-fluoro-4′-α-cyano-5-aza-7, 9-dideaza adenosine as a potent nucleoside inhibitor of respiratory syncytial virus with excellent selectivity over mitochondrial RNA and DNA polymerases. Bioorganic & Medicinal Chemistry Letters. 2015;**25**(12):2484-2487

[27] Deval J, Hong J, Wang G, Taylor J, Smith LK, Fung A, et al. Molecular basis for the selective inhibition of respiratory syncytial virus RNA polymerase by 2′-fluoro-4′-chloromethyl-cytidine

triphosphate. PLoS Pathogens. 2015;**11**(6):e1004995

[28] Wang G, Deval J, Hong J, Dyatkina N, Prhavc M, Taylor J, et al. Discovery of 4′-chloromethyl-2′-deoxy-3′, 5′-di-O-isobutyryl-2′-fluorocytidine (ALS-8176), a first-in-class RSV polymerase inhibitor for treatment of human respiratory syncytial virus infection. Journal of Medicinal Chemistry. 2015;**58**(4):1862-1878

[29] Fix J, Galloux M, Blondot M-L, Eléouët J-F. The insertion of fluorescent proteins in a variable region of respiratory syncytial virus L polymerase results in fluorescent and functional enzymes but with reduced activities. The open virology journal. 2011;**5**:103

[30] Sutto-Ortiz P, Tcherniuk S, Ysebaert N, Abeywickrema P, Noël M, Decombe A, et al. The methyltransferase domain of the respiratory syncytial virus L protein catalyzes cap N7 and 2'-O-methylation. PLoS Pathogens. 2021;**17**(5):e1009562

[31] SnA E, Paris G, de Prat-Gay G. Modular unfolding and dissociation of the human respiratory syncytial virus phosphoprotein P and its interaction with the M2-1 antiterminator: A singular tetramer–tetramer interface arrangement. Biochemistry. 2012;**51**(41):8100-8110

[32] Mazumder B, Barik S. Requirement of casein kinase II-mediated phosphorylation for the transcriptional activity of human respiratory syncytial viral phosphoprotein P: Transdominant negative phenotype of phosphorylation-defective P mutants. Virology. 1994;**205**(1):104-111

[33] Asenjo A, Villanueva N. Regulated but not constitutive human respiratory syncytial virus (HRSV) P protein phosphorylation is essential for oligomerization. FEBS Letters. 2000;**467**(2-3):279-284

[34] Llorente MT, Taylor IA, López-Viñas E, Gomez-Puertas P, Calder LJ, García-Barreno B, et al. Structural properties of the human respiratory syncytial virus P protein: Evidence for an elongated homotetrameric molecule that is the smallest orthologue within the family of paramyxovirus polymerase cofactors. Proteins: Structure, Function, and Bioinformatics. 2008;**72**(3):946-958

[35] Llorente MT, García-Barreno B, Calero M, Camafeita E, Lopez JA, Longhi S, et al. Structural analysis of the human respiratory syncytial virus phosphoprotein: Characterization of an α-helical domain involved in oligomerization. Journal of General Virology. 2006;**87**(1):159-169

[36] Blondot M-L, Dubosclard V, Fix J, Lassoued S, Aumont-Nicaise M, Bontems F, et al. Structure and functional analysis of the RNA-and viral phosphoprotein-binding domain of respiratory syncytial virus M2-1 protein. PLoS Pathogens. 2012;**8**(5):e1002734

[37] Galloux M, Gabiane G, Sourimant J, Richard C-A, England P, Moudjou M, et al. Identification and characterization of the binding site of the respiratory syncytial virus phosphoprotein to RNA-free nucleoprotein. Journal of Virology. 2015;**89**(7):3484-3496

[38] Beavis AC, Tran KC, Barrozo ER, Phan SI, Teng MN, He B. Respiratory syncytial virus phosphoprotein residue S156 plays a role in regulating genome transcription and replication. Journal of Virology. 2021;**95**(24):e01206-e01221

[39] Bukreyev A, Whitehead SS, Murphy BR, Collins PL. Recombinant

respiratory syncytial virus from which the entire SH gene has been deleted grows efficiently in cell culture and exhibits site-specific attenuation in the respiratory tract of the mouse. Journal of Virology. 1997;**71**(12):8973-8982

[40] Rixon HWM, Brown G, Aitken J, McDonald T, Graham S, Sugrue RJ. The small hydrophobic (SH) protein accumulates within lipid-raft structures of the Golgi complex during respiratory syncytial virus infection. Journal of General Virology. 2004;**85**(5):1153-1165

[41] Oomens AG, Bevis KP, Wertz GW. The cytoplasmic tail of the human respiratory syncytial virus F protein plays critical roles in cellular localization of the F protein and infectious progeny production. Journal of Virology. 2006;**80**(21):10465-10477

[42] Collins PL, Huang YT, Wertz GW. Nucleotide sequence of the gene encoding the fusion (F) glycoprotein of human respiratory syncytial virus. Proceedings of the National Academy of Sciences. 1984;**81**(24):7683-7687

[43] Zimmer G, Budz L, Herrler G. Proteolytic activation of respiratory syncytial virus fusion protein: Cleavage at two furin consensus sequences. Journal of Biological Chemistry. 2001;**276**(34):31642-31650

[44] González-Reyes L, Ruiz-Argüello MB, García-Barreno B, Calder L, López JA, Albar JP, et al. Cleavage of the human respiratory syncytial virus fusion protein at two distinct sites is required for activation of membrane fusion. Proceedings of the National Academy of Sciences. 2001;**98**(17):9859-9864

[45] Ghildyal R, Jans A, D, G Bardin P, Mills J. Protein-protein interactions in RSV assembly: Potential targets for attenuating RSV strains. Infectious Disorders-Drug Targets (Formerly Current Drug Targets-Infectious Disorders). 2012;**12**(2):103-109

[46] Bolt G, Pedersen LØ, Birkeslund HH. Cleavage of the respiratory syncytial virus fusion protein is required for its surface expression: Role of furin. Virus Research. 2000;**68**(1):25-33

[47] Day ND, Branigan PJ, Liu C, Gutshall LL, Luo J, Melero JA, et al. Contribution of cysteine residues in the extracellular domain of the F protein of human respiratory syncytial virus to its function. Virology Journal. 2006;**3**(1):1-11

[48] McLellan JS, Chen M, Leung S, Graepel KW, Du X, Yang Y, et al. Structure of RSV fusion glycoprotein trimer bound to a prefusion-specific neutralizing antibody. Science. 2013;**340**(6136):1113-1117

[49] Killikelly AM, Kanekiyo M, Graham BS. Pre-fusion F is absent on the surface of formalin-inactivated respiratory syncytial virus. Scientific Reports. 2016;**6**(1):1-7

[50] McLellan JS, Yang Y, Graham BS, Kwong PD. Structure of respiratory syncytial virus fusion glycoprotein in the postfusion conformation reveals preservation of neutralizing epitopes. Journal of Virology. 2011;**85**(15):7788-7796

[51] Swanson KA, Settembre EC, Shaw CA, Dey AK, Rappuoli R, Mandl CW, et al. Structural basis for immunization with postfusion respiratory syncytial virus fusion F glycoprotein (RSV F) to elicit high neutralizing antibody titers. Proceedings of the National Academy of Sciences. 2011;**108**(23):9619-9624

[52] Battles MB, McLellan JS. Respiratory syncytial virus entry and how to block it. Nature Reviews Microbiology. 2019;**17**(4):233-245

[53] Hendricks DA, Baradaran K, McIntosh K, Patterson JL. Appearance of a soluble form of the G protein of respiratory syncytial virus in fluids of infected cells. Journal of General Virology. 1987;**68**(6):1705-1714

[54] Levine S, Klaiber-Franco R, Paradiso P. Demonstration that glycoprotein G is the attachment protein of respiratory syncytial virus. Journal of General Virology. 1987;**68**(9):2521-2524

[55] Wertz GW, Collins PL, Huang Y, Gruber C, Levine S, Ball LA. Nucleotide sequence of the G protein gene of human respiratory syncytial virus reveals an unusual type of viral membrane protein. Proceedings of the National Academy of Sciences. 1985;**82**(12):4075-4079

[56] Collins PL, Mottet G. Oligomerization and post-translational processing of glycoprotein G of human respiratory syncytial virus: Altered O-glycosylation in the presence of brefeldin A. Journal of General Virology. 1992;**73**(4):849-863

[57] Satake M, Coligan JE, Elango N, Norrby E, Venkatesan S. Respiratory syncytial virus envelope glycoprotein (G) has a novel structure. Nucleic Acids Research. 1985;**13**(21):7795-7812

[58] Sullender WM. Respiratory syncytial virus genetic and antigenic diversity. Clinical Microbiology Reviews. 2000;**13**(1):1-15

[59] Johnson TR, Johnson JE, Roberts SR, Wertz GW, Parker RA, Graham BS. Priming with secreted glycoprotein G of respiratory syncytial virus (RSV) augments interleukin-5 production and tissue eosinophilia after RSV challenge. Journal of Virology. 1998;**72**(4):2871-2880

[60] Kapikian AZ, Mitchell RH, Chanock RM, Shvedoff RA, Stewart CE. An epidemiologic study of altered clinical reactivity to respiratory syncytial (RS) virus infection in children previously vaccinated with an inactivated RS virus vaccine. American Journal of Epidemiology. 1969;**89**(4):405-421

[61] Åkerlind-Stopner B, Hu A, Mufson M, Utter G, Norrby E. Antibody responses of children to the C-terminal peptide of the SH protein of respiratory syncytial virus and the immunological characterization of this protein. Journal of Medical Virology. 1993;**40**(2):112-120

[62] Olmsted RA, Collins PL. The 1A protein of respiratory syncytial virus is an integral membrane protein present as multiple, structurally distinct species. Journal of Virology. 1989;**63**(5):2019-2029

[63] Techaarpornkul S, Barretto N, Peeples ME. Functional analysis of recombinant respiratory syncytial virus deletion mutants lacking the small hydrophobic and/or attachment glycoprotein gene. Journal of Virology. 2001;**75**(15):6825-6834

[64] Heminway B, Yu Y, Tanaka Y, Perrine K, Gustafson E, Bernstein J, et al. Analysis of respiratory syncytial virus F, G, and SH proteins in cell fusion. Virology. 1994;**200**(2):801-805

[65] Feldman S, Crim R, Audet S, Beeler J. Human respiratory syncytial virus surface glycoproteins F, G and SH form an oligomeric complex. Archives of Virology. 2001;**146**(12):2369-2383

[66] Jin H, Zhou H, Cheng X, Tang R, Munoz M, Nguyen N. Recombinant

respiratory syncytial viruses with deletions in the NS1, NS2, SH, and M2-2 genes are attenuated in vitro and in vivo. Virology. 2000;**273**(1):210-218

[67] Gan S-W, Tan E, Lin X, Yu D, Wang J, Tan GM-Y, et al. The small hydrophobic protein of the human respiratory syncytial virus forms pentameric ion channels. Journal of Biological Chemistry. 2012;**287**(29):24671-24689

[68] Triantafilou K, Kar S, Vakakis E, Kotecha S, Triantafilou M. Human respiratory syncytial virus viroporin SH: A viral recognition pathway used by the host to signal inflammasome activation. Thorax. 2013;**68**(1):66-75

[69] Shen C, Zhang Z, Xie T, Ji J, Xu J, Lin L, et al. Rhein suppresses lung inflammatory injury induced by human respiratory syncytial virus through inhibiting NLRP3 inflammasome activation via NF-κB pathway in mice. Frontiers in Pharmacology. 2020;**10**:1600

[70] Fuentes S, Tran KC, Luthra P, Teng MN, He B. Function of the respiratory syncytial virus small hydrophobic protein. Journal of Virology. 2007;**81**(15):8361-8366

[71] Latiff K, Meanger J, Mills J, Ghildyal R. Sequence and structure relatedness of matrix protein of human respiratory syncytial virus with matrix proteins of other negative-sense RNA viruses. Clinical Microbiology and Infection. 2004;**10**(10):945-948

[72] Li D, Jans DA, Bardin PG, Meanger J, Mills J, Ghildyal R. Association of respiratory syncytial virus M protein with viral nucleocapsids is mediated by the M2-1 protein. Journal of Virology. 2008;**82**(17):8863-8870

[73] Marty A, Meanger J, Mills J, Shields B, Ghildyal R. Association of matrix protein of respiratory syncytial virus with the host cell membrane of infected cells. Archives of Virology. 2003;**149**(1):199-210

[74] Ghildyal R, Ho A, Jans DA. Central role of the respiratory syncytial virus matrix protein in infection. FEMS Microbiology Reviews. 2006;**30**(5):692-705

[75] Peeples ME. Paramyxovirus M proteins. The paramyxoviruses: Springer; 1991. pp. 427-456

[76] Ghildyal R, Baulch-Brown C, Mills J, Meanger J. The matrix protein of human respiratory syncytial virus localises to the nucleus of infected cells and inhibits transcription. Archives of Virology. 2003;**148**(7):1419-1429

[77] Ghildyal R, Mills J, Murray M, Vardaxis N, Meanger J. Respiratory syncytial virus matrix protein associates with nucleocapsids in infected cells. Journal of General Virology. 2002;**83**(4):753-757

[78] Ghildyal R, Ho A, Dias M, Soegiyono L, Bardin PG, Tran KC, et al. The respiratory syncytial virus matrix protein possesses a Crm1-mediated nuclear export mechanism. Journal of Virology. 2009;**83**(11):5353-5362

[79] Collins PL, Hill MG, Cristina J, Grosfeld H. Transcription elongation factor of respiratory syncytial virus, a nonsegmented negative-strand RNA virus. Proceedings of the National Academy of Sciences. 1996;**93**(1):81-85

[80] Bermingham A, Collins PL. The M2-2 protein of human respiratory syncytial virus is a regulatory factor involved in the balance between RNA replication and transcription. Proceedings of the National Academy of Sciences. 1999;**96**(20):11259-11264

[81] Tanner SJ, Ariza A, Richard C-A, Kyle HF, Dods RL, Blondot M-L, et al. Crystal structure of the essential transcription antiterminator M2-1 protein of human respiratory syncytial virus and implications of its phosphorylation. Proceedings of the National Academy of Sciences. 2014;**111**(4):1580-1585

[82] Hardy RW, Wertz GW. The product of the respiratory syncytial virus M2 gene ORF1 enhances readthrough of intergenic junctions during viral transcription. Journal of Virology. 1998;**72**(1):520-526

[83] Fearns R, Collins PL. Role of the M2-1 transcription antitermination protein of respiratory syncytial virus in sequential transcription. Journal of Virology. 1999;**73**(7):5852-5864

[84] Teng MN, Whitehead SS, Bermingham A, St. Claire M, Elkins WR, Murphy BR, et al. Recombinant respiratory syncytial virus that does not express the NS1 or M2-2 protein is highly attenuated and immunogenic in chimpanzees. Journal of Virology 2000;74(19):9317-9321.

[85] Boyoglu-Barnum S, Chirkova T, Anderson LJ. Biology of infection and disease pathogenesis to guide RSV vaccine development. Frontiers in Immunology. 2019;**10**:1675

[86] Sedeyn K, Schepens B, Saelens X. Respiratory syncytial virus nonstructural proteins 1 and 2: Exceptional disrupters of innate immune responses. PLoS Pathogens. 2019;**15**(10):e1007984

[87] Spann KM, Tran K-C, Chi B, Rabin RL, Collins PL. Suppression of the induction of alpha, beta, and gamma interferons by the NS1 and NS2 proteins of human respiratory syncytial virus in human epithelial cells and macrophages. Journal of Virology. 2004;**78**(8):4363-4369

[88] Ren J, Liu T, Pang L, Li K, Garofalo RP, Casola A, et al. A novel mechanism for the inhibition of interferon regulatory factor-3-dependent gene expression by human respiratory syncytial virus NS1 protein. The Journal of General Virology. 2011;**92**(Pt 9):2153

[89] Brisse M, Ly H. Comparative structure and function analysis of the RIG-I-like receptors: RIG-I and MDA5. Frontiers in Immunology. 2019;**10**:1586

[90] Spann KM, Tran KC, Collins PL. Effects of nonstructural proteins NS1 and NS2 of human respiratory syncytial virus on interferon regulatory factor 3, NF-κB, and proinflammatory cytokines. Journal of Virology. 2005;**79**(9):5353-5362

[91] Martín-Vicente M, Medrano LM, Resino S, García-Sastre A, Martínez I. TRIM25 in the regulation of the antiviral innate immunity. Frontiers in Immunology. 2017;**8**:1187

[92] Ban J, Lee N-R, Lee N-J, Lee JK, Quan F-S, Inn K-S. Human respiratory syncytial virus NS 1 targets TRIM25 to suppress RIG-I ubiquitination and subsequent RIG-I-mediated antiviral signaling. Viruses. 2018;**10**(12):716

[93] Pei J, Beri NR, Zou AJ, Hubel P, Dorando HK, Bergant V, et al. Nuclear-localized human respiratory syncytial virus NS1 protein modulates host gene transcription. Cell Reports. 2021;**37**(2):109803

[94] Boyapalle S, Wong T, Garay J, Teng M, San Juan-Vergara H, Mohapatra S, et al. Respiratory syncytial virus NS1 protein colocalizes with mitochondrial antiviral signaling protein MAVS following infection. PLoS One. 2012;**7**(2):e29386

[95] Zhang Y, Yang L, Wang H, Zhang G, Sun X. Respiratory syncytial

virus non-structural protein 1 facilitates virus replication through miR-29a-mediated inhibition of interferon-α receptor. Biochemical and Biophysical Research Communications. 2016;**478**(3):1436-1441

[96] Han B, Wang Y, Zheng M. Inhibition of autophagy promotes human RSV NS1-induced inflammation and apoptosis in vitro. Experimental and Therapeutic Medicine. 2021;**22**(4):1-9

[97] Munir S, Le Nouen C, Luongo C, Buchholz UJ, Collins PL, Bukreyev A. Nonstructural proteins 1 and 2 of respiratory syncytial virus suppress maturation of human dendritic cells. Journal of Virology. 2008;**82**(17):8780-8796

[98] Xie J, Long X, Gao L, Chen S, Zhao K, Li W, et al. Respiratory syncytial virus nonstructural protein 1 blocks glucocorticoid receptor nuclear translocation by targeting IPO13 and may account for glucocorticoid insensitivity. The Journal of Infectious Diseases. 2018;**217**(1):35-46

[99] Pei J, Wagner ND, Zou AJ, Chatterjee S, Borek D, Cole AR, et al. Structural basis for IFN antagonism by human respiratory syncytial virus nonstructural protein 2. Proceedings of the National Academy of Sciences. 2021;**118**(10):1-12

[100] Teng MN, Collins PL. Identification of the respiratory syncytial virus proteins required for formation and passage of helper-dependent infectious particles. Journal of Virology. 1998;**72**(7):5707-5716

[101] Kotelkin A, Belyakov IM, Yang L, Berzofsky JA, Collins PL, Bukreyev A. The NS2 protein of human respiratory syncytial virus suppresses the cytotoxic T-cell response as a consequence of suppressing the type I interferon response. Journal of Virology. 2006;**80**(12):5958-5967

[102] Bitko V, Shulyayeva O, Mazumder B, Musiyenko A, Ramaswamy M, Look DC, et al. Nonstructural proteins of respiratory syncytial virus suppress premature apoptosis by an NF-κB-dependent, interferon-independent mechanism and facilitate virus growth. Journal of Virology. 2007;**81**(4):1786-1795

[103] Liesman RM, Buchholz UJ, Luongo CL, Yang L, Proia AD, DeVincenzo JP, et al. RSV-encoded NS2 promotes epithelial cell shedding and distal airway obstruction. The Journal of Clinical Investigation. 2014;**124**(5):2219-2233

[104] Johnson JE, Gonzales RA, Olson SJ, Wright PF, Graham BS. The histopathology of fatal untreated human respiratory syncytial virus infection. Modern Pathology. 2007;**20**(1):108-119

[105] Xu L, Gao H, Zeng J, Liu J, Lu C, Guan X, et al. A fatal case associated with respiratory syncytial virus infection in a young child. BMC Infectious Diseases. 2018;**18**(1):1-7

[106] Pitkäranta A, Virolainen A, Jero J, Arruda E, Hayden FG. Detection of rhinovirus, respiratory syncytial virus, and coronavirus infections in acute otitis media by reverse transcriptase polymerase chain reaction. Pediatrics. 1998;**102**(2):291-295

[107] Rohwedder A, Keminer O, Forster J, Schneider K, Schneider E, Werchau H. Detection of respiratory syncytial virus RNA in blood of neonates by polymerase chain reaction. Journal of Medical Virology. 1998;**54**(4):320-327

[108] Escribano-Romero E, Rawling J, García-Barreno B, Melero JA. The soluble form of human respiratory syncytial

virus attachment protein differs from the membrane-bound form in its oligomeric state but is still capable of binding to cell surface proteoglycans. Journal of Virology. 2004;**78**(7):3524-3532

[109] Krusat T, Streckert H-J. Heparin-dependent attachment ofrespiratory syncytial virus (RSV) to host cells. Archives of Virology. 1997;**142**(6):1247-1254

[110] Feldman SA, Hendry RM, Beeler JA. Identification of a linear heparin binding domain for human respiratory syncytial virus attachment glycoprotein G. Journal of Virology. 1999;**73**(8):6610-6617

[111] Hallak LK, Spillmann D, Collins PL, Peeples ME. Glycosaminoglycan sulfation requirements for respiratory syncytial virus infection. Journal of Virology. 2000;**74**(22):10508-10513

[112] Martínez I, Melero JA. Binding of human respiratory syncytial virus to cells: Implication of sulfated cell surface proteoglycans. Journal of General Virology. 2000;**81**(11):2715-2722

[113] Hallak LK, Collins PL, Knudson W, Peeples ME. Iduronic acid-containing glycosaminoglycans on target cells are required for efficient respiratory syncytial virus infection. Virology. 2000;**271**(2):264-275

[114] Teng MN, Collins PL. The central conserved cystine noose of the attachment G protein of human respiratory syncytial virus is not required for efficient viral infection in vitro or in vivo. Journal of Virology. 2002;**76**(12):6164-6171

[115] Widjojoatmodjo MN, Boes J, van Bers M, van Remmerden Y, Roholl PJ, Luytjes W. A highly attenuated recombinant human respiratory syncytial virus lacking the G protein induces long-lasting protection in cotton rats. Virology Journal. 2010;**7**(1):1-10

[116] Zhang L, Bukreyev A, Thompson CI, Watson B, Peeples ME, Collins PL, et al. Infection of ciliated cells by human parainfluenza virus type 3 in an in vitro model of human airway epithelium. Journal of Virology. 2005;**79**(2):1113-1124

[117] Johnson SM, McNally BA, Ioannidis I, Flano E, Teng MN, Oomens AG, et al. Respiratory syncytial virus uses CX3CR1 as a receptor on primary human airway epithelial cultures. PLoS Pathogens. 2015;**11**(12):e1005318

[118] Tripp RA, Jones LP, Haynes LM, Zheng H, Murphy PM, Anderson LJ. CX3C chemokine mimicry by respiratory syncytial virus G glycoprotein. Nature Immunology. 2001;**2**(8):732-738

[119] Ha B, Chirkova T, Boukhvalova MS, Sun HY, Walsh EE, Anderson CS, et al. Mutation of respiratory syncytial virus G protein's CX3C motif attenuates infection in cotton rats and primary human airway epithelial cells. Vaccine. 2019;**7**(3):69

[120] Lee H-J, Lee J-Y, Park M-H, Kim J-Y, Chang J. Monoclonal antibody against G glycoprotein increases respiratory syncytial virus clearance in vivo and prevents vaccine-enhanced diseases. PLoS One. 2017;**12**(1):e0169139

[121] Jeong K-I, Piepenhagen PA, Kishko M, DiNapoli JM, Groppo RP, Zhang L, et al. CX3CR1 is expressed in differentiated human ciliated airway cells and co-localizes with respiratory syncytial virus on cilia in a G protein-dependent manner. PLoS One. 2015;**10**(6):e0130517

[122] Karron RA, Buonagurio DA, Georgiu AF, Whitehead SS, Adamus JE,

Clements-Mann ML, et al. Respiratory syncytial virus (RSV) SH and G proteins are not essential for viral replication in vitro: Clinical evaluation and molecular characterization of a cold-passaged, attenuated RSV subgroup B mutant. Proceedings of the National Academy of Sciences. 1997;**94**(25):13961-13966

[123] Feldman SA, Audet S, Beeler JA. The fusion glycoprotein of human respiratory syncytial virus facilitates virus attachment and infectivity via an interaction with cellular heparan sulfate. Journal of Virology. 2000;**74**(14):6442-6447

[124] Behera AK, Matsuse H, Kumar M, Kong X, Lockey RF, Mohapatra SS. Blocking intercellular adhesion molecule-1 on human epithelial cells decreases respiratory syncytial virus infection. Biochemical and Biophysical Research Communications. 2001;**280**(1):188-195

[125] Currier MG, Lee S, Stobart CC, Hotard AL, Villenave R, Meng J, et al. EGFR interacts with the fusion protein of respiratory syncytial virus strain 2-20 and mediates infection and mucin expression. PLoS Pathogens. 2016;**12**(5):e1005622

[126] Tayyari F, Marchant D, Moraes TJ, Duan W, Mastrangelo P, Hegele RG. Identification of nucleolin as a cellular receptor for human respiratory syncytial virus. Nature Medicine. 2011;**17**(9):1132-1135

[127] Griffiths CD, Bilawchuk LM, McDonough JE, Jamieson KC, Elawar F, Cen Y, et al. IGF1R is an entry receptor for respiratory syncytial virus. Nature. 2020;**583**(7817):615-619

[128] Srinivasakumar N, Ogra P, Flanagan T. Characteristics of fusion of respiratory syncytial virus with HEp-2 cells as measured by R18 fluorescence dequenching assay. Journal of Virology. 1991;**65**(8):4063-4069

[129] Kahn JS, Schnell MJ, Buonocore L, Rose JK. Recombinant vesicular stomatitis virus expressing respiratory syncytial virus (RSV) glycoproteins: RSV fusion protein can mediate infection and cell fusion. Virology. 1999;**254**(1):81-91

[130] Krzyzaniak MA, Zumstein MT, Gerez JA, Picotti P, Helenius A. Host cell entry of respiratory syncytial virus involves macropinocytosis followed by proteolytic activation of the F protein. PLoS Pathogens. 2013;**9**(4):e1003309

[131] Carromeu C, Simabuco F, Tamura R, Arcieri LF, Ventura A. Intracellular localization of human respiratory syncytial virus L protein. Archives of Virology. 2007;**152**(12):2259-2263

[132] Fearns R, Deval J. New antiviral approaches for respiratory syncytial virus and other mononegaviruses: Inhibiting the RNA polymerase. Antiviral Research. 2016;**134**:63-76

[133] García J, García-Barreno B, Vivo A, Melero JA. Cytoplasmic inclusions of respiratory syncytial virus-infected cells: Formation of inclusion bodies in transfected cells that coexpress the nucleoprotein, the phosphoprotein, and the 22K protein. Virology. 1993;**195**(1):243-247

[134] Norrby E, Marusyk H, Örvell C. Morphogenesis of respiratory syncytial virus in a green monkey kidney cell line (Vero). Journal of Virology. 1970;**6**(2):237-242

[135] García-Barreno B, Delgado T, Melero JA. Identification of protein regions involved in the interaction of human respiratory syncytial virus

phosphoprotein and nucleoprotein: Significance for nucleocapsid assembly and formation of cytoplasmic inclusions. Journal of Virology. 1996;**70**(2):801-808

[136] Richard C-A, Rincheval V, Lassoued S, Fix J, Cardone C, Esneau C, et al. RSV hijacks cellular protein phosphatase 1 to regulate M2-1 phosphorylation and viral transcription. PLoS Pathogens. 2018;**14**(3):e1006920

[137] Bajorek M, Galloux M, Richard C-A, Szekely O, Rosenzweig R, Sizun C, et al. Tetramerization of phosphoprotein is essential for respiratory syncytial virus budding while its N-terminal region mediates direct interactions with the matrix protein. Journal of Virology. 2021;**95**(7):e02217-e02220

[138] Mitra R, Baviskar P, Duncan-Decocq RR, Patel D, Oomens AG. The human respiratory syncytial virus matrix protein is required for maturation of viral filaments. Journal of Virology. 2012;**86**(8):4432-4443

[139] Santangelo P, Nitin N, LaConte L, Woolums A, Bao G. Live-cell characterization and analysis of a clinical isolate of bovine respiratory syncytial virus, using molecular beacons. Journal of Virology. 2006;**80**(2):682-688

[140] Lindquist ME, Lifland AW, Utley TJ, Santangelo PJ, Crowe JE Jr. Respiratory syncytial virus induces host RNA stress granules to facilitate viral replication. Journal of Virology. 2010;**84**(23):12274-12284

[141] Fearns R, Peeples ME, Collins PL. Mapping the transcription and replication promoters of respiratory syncytial virus. Journal of Virology. 2002;**76**(4):1663-1672

[142] Collins PL, Mink MA, Stec DS. Rescue of synthetic analogs of respiratory syncytial virus genomic RNA and effect of truncations and mutations on the expression of a foreign reporter gene. Proceedings of the National Academy of Sciences. 1991;**88**(21):9663-9667

[143] Mink MA, Stec DS, Collins PL. Nucleotide sequences of the 3′ leader and 5′ trailer regions of human respiratory syncytial virus genomic RNA. Virology. 1991;**185**(2):615-624

[144] Kuo L, Grosfeld H, Cristina J, Hill MG, Collins PL. Effects of mutations in the gene-start and gene-end sequence motifs on transcription of monocistronic and dicistronic minigenomes of respiratory syncytial virus. Journal of Virology. 1996;**70**(10):6892-6901

[145] Tremaglio CZ, Noton SL, Deflubé LR, Fearns R. Respiratory syncytial virus polymerase can initiate transcription from position 3 of the leader promoter. Journal of Virology. 2013;**87**(6):3196-3207

[146] Kuo L, Fearns R, Collins PL. The structurally diverse intergenic regions of respiratory syncytial virus do not modulate sequential transcription by a dicistronic minigenome. Journal of Virology. 1996;**70**(9):6143-6150

[147] Liuzzi M, Mason SW, Cartier M, Lawetz C, McCollum RS, Dansereau N, et al. Inhibitors of respiratory syncytial virus replication target cotranscriptional mRNA guanylylation by viral RNA-dependent RNA polymerase. Journal of Virology. 2005;**79**(20):13105-13115

[148] Gubbay O, Curran J, Kolakofsky D. Sendai virus genome synthesis and assembly are coupled: A possible mechanism to promote viral RNA polymerase processivity. Journal of General Virology. 2001;**82**(12):2895-2903

[149] McGivern DR, Collins PL, Fearns R. Identification of internal sequences

in the 3′ leader region of human respiratory syncytial virus that enhance transcription and confer replication processivity. Journal of Virology. 2005;**79**(4):2449-2460

[150] Peeples ME, Collins PL. Mutations in the 5′ trailer region of a respiratory syncytial virus minigenome which limit RNA replication to one step. Journal of Virology. 2000;**74**(1):146-155

[151] Noton SL, Deflubé LR, Tremaglio CZ, Fearns R. The respiratory syncytial virus polymerase has multiple RNA synthesis activities at the promoter. 2012 PLoS Pathogens. 2012;**8**(10): e1002980

[152] Noton SL, Cowton VM, Zack CR, McGivern DR, Fearns R. Evidence that the polymerase of respiratory syncytial virus initiates RNA replication in a nontemplated fashion. Proceedings of the National Academy of Sciences. 2010;**107**(22):10226-10231

[153] Hanley LL, McGivern DR, Teng MN, Djang R, Collins PL, Fearns R. Roles of the respiratory syncytial virus trailer region: Effects of mutations on genome production and stress granule formation. Virology. 2010;**406**(2):241-252

[154] Cressey TN, Noton SL, Nagendra K, Braun MR, Fearns R. Mechanism for de novo initiation at two sites in the respiratory syncytial virus promoter. Nucleic Acids Research. 2018;**46**(13):6785-6796

[155] Grosfeld H, Hill MG, Collins PL. RNA replication by respiratory syncytial virus (RSV) is directed by the N, P, and L proteins; transcription also occurs under these conditions but requires RSV superinfection for efficient synthesis of full-length mRNA. Journal of Virology. 1995;**69**(9):5677-5686

[156] Roberts SR, Compans RW, Wertz GW. Respiratory syncytial virus matures at the apical surfaces of polarized epithelial cells. Journal of Virology. 1995;**69**(4):2667-2673

[157] Brown G, Aitken J, Rixon HWM, Sugrue RJ. Caveolin-1 is incorporated into mature respiratory syncytial virus particles during virus assembly on the surface of virus-infected cells. Journal of General Virology. 2002;**83**(3):611-621

[158] Brown G, Rixon HWM, Sugrue RJ. Respiratory syncytial virus assembly occurs in GM1-rich regions of the host-cell membrane and alters the cellular distribution of tyrosine phosphorylated caveolin-1. Journal of General Virology. 2002;**83**(8):1841-1850

[159] Simons K. Ikonen E. Functional rafts in cell membranes. nature. 1997;**387**(6633):569-572

[160] Shaikh FY, Utley TJ, Craven RE, Rogers MC, Lapierre LA, Goldenring JR, et al. Respiratory syncytial virus assembles into structured filamentous virion particles independently of host cytoskeleton and related proteins. PLoS One. 2012;**7**(7):e40826

[161] Baviskar PS, Hotard AL, Moore ML, Oomens AG. The respiratory syncytial virus fusion protein targets to the perimeter of inclusion bodies and facilitates filament formation by a cytoplasmic tail-dependent mechanism. Journal of Virology. 2013;**87**(19):10730-10741

[162] McCurdy LH, Graham BS. Role of plasma membrane lipid microdomains in respiratory syncytial virus filament formation. Journal of Virology. 2003;**77**(3):1747-1756

[163] Gower TL, Pastey MK, Peeples ME, Collins PL, McCurdy LH, Hart TK, et al.

RhoA signaling is required for respiratory syncytial virus-induced syncytium formation and filamentous virion morphology. Journal of Virology. 2005;**79**(9):5326-5336

[164] Jeffree CE, Brown G, Aitken J, Su-Yin DY, Tan B-H, Sugrue RJ. Ultrastructural analysis of the interaction between F-actin and respiratory syncytial virus during virus assembly. Virology. 2007;**369**(2):309-323

[165] Ghildyal R, Ho A, Wagstaff KM, Dias MM, Barton CL, Jans P, et al. Nuclear import of the respiratory syncytial virus matrix protein is mediated by importin β1 independent of importin α. Biochemistry. 2005;**44**(38):12887-12895

[166] Rodríguez L, Cuesta I, Asenjo A, Villanueva N. Human respiratory syncytial virus matrix protein is an RNA-binding protein: Binding properties, location and identity of the RNA contact residues. Journal of General Virology. 2004;**85**(3):709-719

[167] Ghildyal R, Li D, Peroulis I, Shields B, Bardin PG, Teng MN, et al. Interaction between the respiratory syncytial virus G glycoprotein cytoplasmic domain and the matrix protein. Journal of General Virology. 2005;**86**(7):1879-1884

[168] Vanover D, Smith DV, Blanchard EL, Alonas E, Kirschman JL, Lifland AW, et al. RSV glycoprotein and genomic RNA dynamics reveal filament assembly prior to the plasma membrane. Nature Communications. 2017;**8**(1):1-15

[169] Brock SC, Goldenring JR, Crowe JE. Apical recycling systems regulate directional budding of respiratory syncytial virus from polarized epithelial cells. Proceedings of the National Academy of Sciences. 2003;**100**(25):15143-15148

[170] Utley TJ, Ducharme NA, Varthakavi V, Shepherd BE, Santangelo PJ, Lindquist ME, et al. Respiratory syncytial virus uses a Vps4-independent budding mechanism controlled by Rab11-FIP2. Proceedings of the National Academy of Sciences. 2008;**105**(29):10209-10214

[171] Cifuentes-Munoz N, Dutch RE, Cattaneo R. Direct cell-to-cell transmission of respiratory viruses: The fast lanes. PLoS Pathogens. 2018;**14**(6):e1007015

[172] Mehedi M, Collins PL, Buchholz UJ. A novel host factor for human respiratory syncytial virus. Communicative & Integrative Biology. 2017;**10**(3):e1319025

[173] Mehedi M, Smelkinson M, Kabat J, Ganesan S, Collins PL, Buchholz UJ. Multicolor stimulated emission depletion (STED) microscopy to generate high-resolution images of respiratory syncytial virus particles and infected cells. Bio-Protocol. 2017;**7**(17):1-10

[174] Paluck A, Osan J, Hollingsworth L, Talukdar SN, Saegh AA, Mehedi M. Role of ARP2/3 complex-driven actin polymerization in RSV infection. Pathogens. 2021;**11**(1):1-12

Section 2

Influenza Virus

Chapter 3

Influenza Viruses: Targetting Conserved Viral Ha-Stem, Matrix and Nucleo-Proteins to Disarm a Resilient and Recurring Pandemic

Babayemi Olawale Oladejo and Covenant Femi Adeboboye

Abstract

Much to the current worldwide pandemic caused by the SARs-Cov-2 virus, common flu caused by Influenza virus remain a long-standing mayhem to global health. Influenza viruses are important human pathogens responsible for substantial seasonal and pandemic morbidity and mortality. Despite the efficiency of widely available antiviral neuraminidase (NA) inhibitor drugs, and multiple formulations of the influenza vaccines, including inactivated influenza vaccines (IIV); a recombinant inactivated vaccine (RIV); and a live, attenuated influenza vaccine (LAIV), Influenza virus infection still remains an ongoing health and economic burden causing epidemics with pandemic potential keeping scientist on their toes in researching to combat the complexity often associated with the pathogenesis of these viral infection and perhaps its associated genetics. Most recent strides and advances within the global research landscape has seen efforts channeled towards the discovery and production of universal vaccines in a bid to address the unique challenge associated with the multiple viral strain explosion often encountered with influenza viruses. An important strategy for accomplishing this is to provoke an immune response to the virus's "Achille's heel", i.e., conserved viral proteins, through targeting the hemagglutinin (HA) glycoprotein or protein domains shared by seasonal and pre-pandemic strains.

Keywords: influenza virus, ARDS, hemagglutinin, neuraminidase, universal vaccines

1. Introduction

Influenza viruses are RNA viruses that cause infectious respiratory diseases that are majorly characterized by fever, congestion, and myalgia, which ranges in severity from mild to life-threating, and they are estimated to cause about 250,000 to 500,000 deaths globally per year [1]. They are single-stranded, helically shaped, and belongs to the orthomyxovirus family consisting of 5 influenza virus genera, ranging averagely from 80 to 120 nm in size [2]. They often contain 8 gene segments that encodes 11 proteins (**Figure 1**). These segments encode viral proteins including hemagglutinin (HA), neuraminidase (NA), nonstructural 1 (NS1), NS2, matrix 1 (M1), M2,

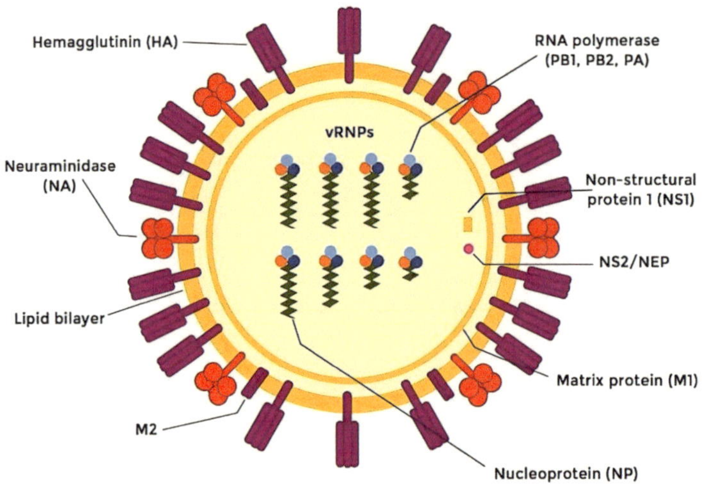

Figure 1.
Showing all the eight gene segments and encoded proteins of influenza A virus. Influenza virus's genome is eight-segmented and encodes for two surface glycoproteins which includes neuraminidase (NA) and hemagglutinin (HA); matrix protein 2 (M2) ion channel that are securely buried into the viral lipid envelope; matrix protein 1 (M1) which lies beneath the membrane; protein-basic protein (PB1, PB2) protein-acidic protein (PA) which makes up the RNA polymerase complex that is associated with the encapsilated genome; nucleoprotein (NP) which coats the viral genome and nonstructural proteins (NS1 and NS2) which suppresses host cell's mRNA production and serves as interferon antagonism.

nucleoprotein (NP), nuclear export protein (NEP), polymerase acid (PA), polymerase basic 1 (PB1) and PB2 [3]. Influenza viruses are uniquely known to express spike glycoproteins such as hemagglutinin (HA) which facilitates viral recognition of host receptor binding site and neuraminidase (NA) which also aids viral release after replication within the host cells [2, 4]. HA binds Sialic acid bonded with galactose, in avian influenza (H5N1) affinity binding occurs with the α-2,3 sialic acid galactose receptor complex of birds in contrast with the α-2,6 binding in human Influenza virus A infections [1, 4, 5].

Till date, three types of influenza virus have been known to cause infection in humans: A, B, and C. Type A influenza has subtypes determined by the surface antigens hemagglutinin (HA) and neuraminidase (NA). There are 18 different H subtypes and 11 different N subtypes. Eight H subtypes (H1, H2, H3, H5, H6, H7, H9, H10) and six N subtypes (N1, N2, N6, N7, N8, and N9) have been detected in humans. Type B influenza is classified into two lineages: B/Yamagata and B/Victoria [2]. Influenza B commonly affects children while Influenza C is rarely reported as a cause of human illness, which is probably because most cases are subclinical. Influenza C has still not been associated with any epidemic disease outbreak so far. WHO currently classifies influenza A(H1N1) and A(H3N2) as circulating seasonal influenza A virus subtypes, while also classifying avian influenza virus subtypes A(H5N1) and A(H9N2) and swine influenza virus subtypes A(H1N1) and (H3N2) as zoonotic or variant influenza [2, 6].

Enormous efforts are currently aimed at preventing and treating influenza infections, including seasonal and pandemic influenza, however, outbreaks still remain a major public health challenge globally [1, 4]. This is majorly due to influenza viruses rapidly undergoing genetic mutations that restrict the long-lasting efficacy of vaccine-induced immune responses and therapeutic regimens [1]. These major viral genetic changes involve Antigenic Drift, which is caused by point mutations in genes encoding HA and N glycoproteins spikes thereby allowing for viral immune invasion against host responses and generated antibodies like vaccines. Similarly, antigenic shift which occurs in influenza virus A, caused by viral genome reassortment/swapping mechanisms among two different subtypes of influenza A which are replicating within the same host causing a jump to new species of host, and a highly diverse structure of virus able to cause the occasional pandemics seen in the world [2]. A combination of antiviral agents and vaccines remains the general prevention and treatment measures for influenza-related morbidity and mortality, however complications arising from viral genetic changes has bolstered scientific efforts on a journey to the discovery of universal vaccines.

2. Pathophysiology

Following respiratory transmission, human influenza virus attaches to and penetrates the respiratory epithelial cells in the trachea and bronchi. Other cell types often affected in the respiratory tract includes several immune cells, which can be infected by the virus and initiate viral protein production. However, the efficiency of replication varies among various affected cell types, and, in humans, the respiratory epithelium is the only site where the hemagglutinin (HA) molecule is effectively cleaved [5, 7]. The primary mechanism of influenza pathophysiology is a result of lung inflammation and compromise that is caused by direct viral infection of the respiratory epithelium, combined with the effects of lung inflammation also caused by immune responses recruited to handle the spread of the virus [7]. Influenza-mediated respiratory tract damage is caused by a combination of events, including: a) intrinsic viral pathogenicity due to its affinity for host airway and alveolar epithelial cells; and b) a robust host innate immune response, which, while aiding in viral clearance, can aggravate the severity of lung injury [7].

The host cell is then destroyed as a result of viral replication. Viremia, or the presence of a virus in the blood, has, on the other hand, is seldomly observed and never widely documented. Virus is released in respiratory secretions for 5 to 10 days, peaking 1 to 3 days after disease start [5, 7]. Inflammation caused by influenza pathogenic events can extend systemically and appear as multiorgan failure, the most common of which are lung compromise and severe respiratory distress [8]. Some links have also been found between influenza virus infection and cardiac complications, such as an increased risk of myocardial illness in the weeks following infection. Beyond the basic inflammatory profile, several of these processes remain uncertain [9, 10]. Researchers find it theoretically helpful to divide the progression of IAV infection into three stages, with the idea that many of these processes occur concurrently throughout the injury. The first is viral infection and replication in the airway and alveolar epithelium, during which methods that restrict viral entrance or replication might prevent or reduce the severity of the infection. The innate immune response to the virus is followed by the adaptive immunological response, which is crucial for viral clearance but may also cause severe damage to the alveolar epithelium and endothelium. The third step is the establishment of long-term immunity to the infecting virus strain, which is followed by the resolution of infiltrates and regeneration of damaged lung tissue, during which time the patient is more vulnerable to secondary bacterial infection [4, 5, 7].

2.1 Acute respiratory distress syndrome

The influenza viruses are significantly important human pathogens. In humans, infection of the lower respiratory tract of can result in flooding of the alveolar compartment, development of acute respiratory distress syndrome and death from respiratory failure. The extent to which the virus infiltrates the lower respiratory tract is an important factor in determining the degree of associated disease complications [8]. Infection of alveolar epithelial cells appears to cause the development of severe illness by damaging important mediators of gas exchange and permitting viral exposure to endothelial cells. Early interactions between the influenza virus, alveolar macrophages in the lung airways, and the epithelial lining are significant determinants of alveolar disease development [9]. Once this delicate barrier is penetrated, cytokine and viral antigen exposure to the endothelium layer can exacerbate inflammation, with endothelial cells being a primary source of pro-inflammatory cytokines that influence the amount and nature of future innate and adaptive immune responses [10].

In the final pathological stages, just like in the SARS-CoV-2 infection, where reports from Lancet on COVID-19 pathogenesis reveals that acute respiratory distress syndrome (ARDS) is the main cause of death in most patients [11–14], influenza virus infection also initiates hypoxia and progression to ARDS [15]. ARDS is majorly experienced as shortness of breath and it's also a common immunopathological event in SARS-CoV and MERS-CoV infections [11]. Clinically, severe Influenza A Virus infection can cause bilateral lung infiltrates and hypoxaemia, which are symptoms of acute respiratory distress syndrome (ARDS), and death from hypoxaemic respiratory failure is a major contributor to mortality [16–21]. The cumulative incidence of ARDS related to seasonal IAV infection has been estimated to be 2.7 cases per 100,000 person-years, accounting for 4% of all respiratory failure hospitalizations throughout the influenza season [22].

2.2 Clinical manifestations and complications

In most cases, influenza produces a simple respiratory illness with a cough, fever, myalgias, chills or sweats, and malaise that lasts two to eight days. The onset is usually quick. Children might have unusual gastrointestinal symptoms such as vomiting and diarrhea. A small percentage of patients, particularly elderly individuals, young children, and those with medical comorbidities, will develop severe illness from viral or secondary bacterial pneumonia, resulting in respiratory and multiorgan failure. Extrapulmonary events are extremely uncommon [23, 24].

Common symptoms such as running nose, sore throat, muscle pains, fever, headaches and fatigue can trigger the release of pro-inflammatory cytokines and chemokines such as tumor necrosis factor or interferon from infected cells might be capable of producing a life-threatening cytokine storm [25]. Influenza does cause tissue damage compared to common cold that is caused by rhinovirus and as such symptoms might not entirely depend on inflammatory response. Also, the large amounts of cytokines have been observed to be dependent on the levels of viral replication produced by the strains [26]. Flu epidemics are difficult to control due to their rapid spread. However, influenza virus has a short generation time of two days (the time from being infected and then to infect the next person). Individuals can become infectious before being symptomatic thus quarantines following noticeable sign and symptom of the infection is not an effective public health intervention [27]. The virus shedding in an average person peak on day two while symptoms becoming apparent on day three [28].

3. Prevention and treatment

Early anti-influenza drugs were synthesized by large scale screening methods without the knowledge of their chemical structures and mechanisms of action [29], whereas, the recent antivirals have been discovered based on the structure of influenza virus protein as drug targets using X-ray crystallography method. This is structure based, involving the use of organic compounds that are able to bind to viral target protein receptors [30]. These structures have high binding affinity to the viral target following chemical synthesis and effective antiviral screening using standard in vitro assays such as cell based antiviral screening [31] and biochemical evaluation [32]. Some cell based antiviral screening includes plaque assays for studying replication in virus, yield-reduction assays for quantifying specific viral antigens and dye uptake for measuring cytopathic effect. The application of bioinformatics, robotics, miniaturization strategies have led to an advanced and high-throughput drug screening of large drug libraries with unique chemical structures [33] and computational screening [34]. In vivo drug screening using various animal models such as chicken, mouse, ferret have been used to evaluate new drugs [35] this is followed by clinical trials to study its bio-safety, kinetics and tolerance in human [36].

Advances has since then seen the treatment of influenza virus infection basically through vaccines, monoclonal antibodies and antivirals drugs. Antiviral influenza drugs are mostly NA inhibitors; however, they generally have short therapeutic window and current show emerging drug resistance [37]. Till date, four (4) antiviral drugs have been approved for the treatment of influenza: the NA inhibitors oseltamivir (Tamifu), peramivir (Rapivab), zanamivir (Relenza), and the cap-dependent endonuclease inhibitor baloxavir (Xofuza) [23, 37]. Oseltamivir is the preferred treatment for patients with severe influenza. Intravenous peramivir is an option for these patients if there are contraindications to or concerns about reduced bioavailability of oral oseltamivir [24]. Baloxavir is preferred for the treatment of uncomplicated influenza in patients of age 12 years and older. A study was conducted to compare baloxavir with oseltamivir and placebo in 1436 healthy people between 12 to 65 years of age who had influenza, baloxavir and oseltamivir reduced symptom duration by approximately one day compared with placebo. Adamantanes (amantadine and rimantadine [Flumadine]) are also approved for influenza treatment but are not currently recommended because these medications are not active against influenza B, and most influenza A strains have shown resistance to adamantane for the past 10 years [24].

Vaccines remain extremely essential to the prevention of the infection. Vaccination is the most preferred method for prevention, and routine chemoprophylaxis within the community is not recommended. The first influenza vaccine was developed in 1945, and since seen several others produced. Multiple formulations of the influenza vaccine are available, including inactivated influenza vaccines (IIV); a recombinant inactivated vaccine (RIV); and a live, attenuated influenza vaccine (LAIV). LAIV shows one of the best efficacies at around 70% and tends to be more effective in children. It delivers more NA and M2 antigens, triggers mucosal responses including IgA, and has the potential for inducing CD8 T cell responses [38].

As a primary prophylactic countermeasure, annual influenza vaccination is engaged globally with the aim of limiting influenza burden. However, the effectiveness of the current available influenza vaccines is limited because they only confer protective immunity when there is antigenic similarity between the selected vaccine strains and circulating influenza isolates. The consequences of antigenic drift or shift, results in an antigenic mismatch between the current vaccines and circulating influenza isolates. Accumulation of mutations, especially at key antigenic sites in the HA globular head, due to the absence of the proofreading activity of the viral RNA polymerase and then to the selective pressure exerted by the host immune system is often responsible for the escape of influenza virus from pre-existing immunity in the case of antigenic drift [39]. There is therefore a crucial need to develop a more effective broadly-reactive (universal) influenza vaccine with the capability to confer protection against both seasonal and newly emerging pre-pandemic strains.

3.1 The journey to a universal flu vaccine

In influenza virus vaccine design, the major targets of the antibody response against the virus are the surface glycoprotein antigens hemagglutinin (HA) and neuraminidase (NA). As earlier stated, Hemagglutinin (HA) and neuraminidase (NA), are the main surface glycoproteins on influenza viral particles. NA is however less abundantly expressed on the virion in comparison HA expression, with HA to NA ratio often ranging from 4:1 to 5:1 [38]. The influenza HA is responsible for binding to sialic acid, the receptor on target host cells, and there are approximately 500 molecules of HA per virion [40]. The mature form of the HA glycoprotein exists as a homotrimer containing three HA monomers that are composed of a globular head and a stem/stalk region. The receptor binding site (RBS) is present in the globular head, which is however a hypervariable region of the protein, while the stem region is majorly involved in the pH-induced fusion event triggered by endosome acidification following viral adsorption. The stem/stalk region of the HA is more conserved among and across HA subtypes belonging to the same group [38]. Antibody response elicited against this stem/stalk region forms one of the major approaches towards developing a more responsive vaccine to both current and future strains of influenza viruses (**Figure 2**).

3.1.1 Stem-based universal vaccine approaches

Influenza virus infection can elicit neutralizing antibodies against both the globular head and the stem structures of the HA viral protein. Currently, ongoing strategies for more efficacious vaccine development is aimed at eliciting antibodies that target the conserved stem region of HA since previously existing influenza vaccines only show minimal induction of stem-directed humoral immunity [3]. Several studies describe ongoing approaches to elicit stem-directed antibodies including sequential immunization with heterologous influenza strains, immunization with modified proteins by removing or glycan-masking the globular head, referred to as headless HA, through minimizing epitopes of the stem region, hyperglycosylated HA head domain, Chimeric HA, and Mosaic HA [3, 38]. Self-reactivity of this antibodies may occur due to their polyreactive profile and the proximity of the HA stem region to the cell membrane which is a crucial limitation described by scientists to this approach.

Nachbagauer et al. [40] recently presented a unique concept in the stem-based approach using the context of a LAIV with a H8 head domain and an H1 stem domain

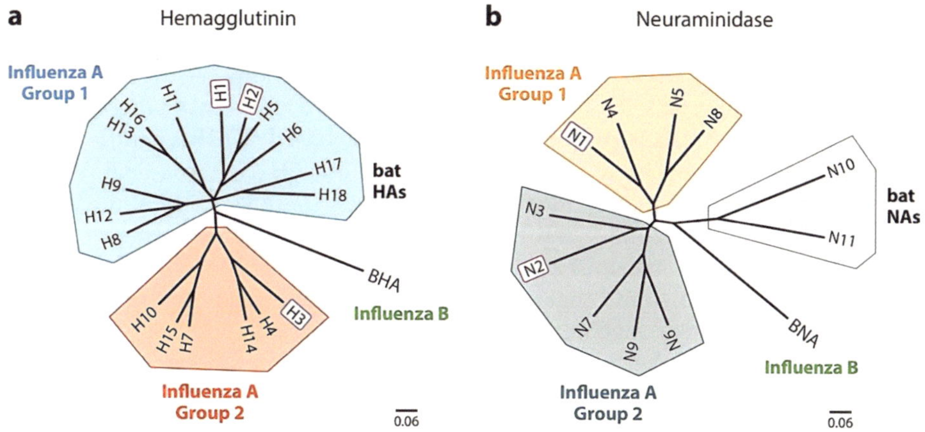

Figure 2.
Showing the phylogenetic trees of (a) hemagglutinin (HA) and (b) neuraminidase (NA). The primary surface glycoproteins of influenza viruses, HA and NA, are divided into several categories and subtypes. During the last century, only viruses producing H1, H2, or H3 HAs and N1 or N2 NAs (such as H1N1, H2N2, or H3N2; circled in purple) have spread widely in the human population. The scale bars represent a 6% change in amino acid levels (source: [41]).

(cH8/1) and a split-inactivated vaccine with an H5 head domain and an H1 stem domain (cH5/1) [40]. Using preclinical ferret investigations, the scientists assessed protection against pandemic H1N1 virus challenge using several sequential prime-boost combinations and vaccination regimens. These studies show that a sequential live-attenuated followed by split-inactivated viral vaccination strategy provides superior protection against pandemic H1N1 infection. Scientists have characterized this notion as a sequential immunization and chimeric HA proteins approach to stem-based universal vaccine design.

Furthermore, in a stem-based immunogens approach to the universal influenza vaccine design, based on the H1 subtype, Impagliazzo et al. created stable mini-HA stem antigens, where the best candidate demonstrated structural and binding characteristics with widely neutralizing antibodies equivalent to full-length HA, indicating correct folding. This immunogen totally protected mice in lethal heterologous and heterosubtypic challenge scenarios and lowered fever in cynomolgus monkeys following a sublethal challenge [42]. However, determining the effectiveness of antibodies targeting conserved epitopes in the HA stem region to offer protection remains a critical challenge [43].

3.1.2 Consensus based approach: computationally optimized broadly reactive antigens (COBRAs)

Furthermore, in order to overcome the extreme variability of influenza HA, in particular at the head region, Giles and Ross, [44] described the generation of computationally optimized broadly reactive antigens (COBRAs) for the influenza HA. The COBRA-based approach is a classic reverse vaccinology approach based on multiple layering of consensus HA protein sequences, followed by the generation of a final consensus sequence capable of recapitulating, in a unique protein, amino acid changes undergone by influenza virus from the past years to the present [45]. In this approach, a phylogenetic tree is inferred using hemagglutinin (HA) amino acid sequences. Primary and secondary consensus sequences are constructed, and the secondary consensus sequences are subsequently aligned to provide the resultant consensus, known as COBRA. In multiple clinical investigations, a firm called Sanofi-Pasteur used this method with a mechanism called Elicite HAI+ antibodies [46–49].

More specifically, vaccination of mice with H1N1-based COBRA candidates resulted in broad HAI activity against a panel of 17 H1N1 virus strains. Furthermore, when inoculated mice were challenged, there was little or no detectable viral replication, as found in animals immunized with a matching approved vaccine [46]. Similarly, previous studies describing the design and generation of H5N1-based COBRA found that mice, ferrets, and nonhuman primates (Cynomolgus macaques) vaccinated with COBRA clade 2 HA H5N1 virus-like particles (VLPs) had higher HAI antibody titers recognizing different isolates representing divergent subclades [44, 49].

Aside from the COBRA-based strategy, there are several potential vaccines targeting the HA head. Song et al. [50] demonstrated the production of a fusion protein comprised of the globular HA head domains (HA1–2, spanning amino acids 62–284) from H7N9 and the Salmonella typhimurium flagellin (fliC) produced in *Escherichia coli* (*E. coli*). The authors chose fliC as a potent Toll-like receptor-5 (TLR5) ligand in order to induce an innate immune response with subsequent induction of cytokine production and dendritic cell activation, ultimately leading to higher titers of antigen-specific IgG recognizing different isolates representing divergent subclades [44, 49].

3.1.3 Vaccines targeting internal viral proteins

Internal influenza virus proteins are often highly conserved, making them viable targets for a universal vaccination. Although these proteins are rarely detected on virions or cell surfaces, making them inaccessible to antibodies, they are abundant in infected cells, where they are also processed and presented to T cells through major histocompatibility complex molecules. T cells have therefore been proven to play a significant role in influenza virus immunity. In this approach, NP and M1 have been widely studied as possible targets for universal T cell–based vaccine. Virus-based and DNA vaccination approaches have been shown in animal models to induce protective immune responses, and they are now being studied in a variety of clinical trials [41]. Over two consecutive influenza seasons, Evans et al. [51] conducted a phase 2b, randomized, placebo-controlled, double-blind trial of a recombinant viral-vectored vaccine (modified vaccinia Ankara expressing virus nucleoprotein and matrix protein 1; MVA-NP + M1), which has been shown to induce both CD4 and CD8 T cells, at eight outpatient clinical trial sites in Australia. They wanted to see if generating extra responses to conserved CD4 and CD8 T-cell antigens improves routine influenza vaccination. Based on their findings, they concluded that MVA-NP + M1 was well tolerated, with no vaccine-related major side effects. When administered within 28 days of normal QIV immunization, a vaccine intended to stimulate modest T-cell responses to cross-reactive internal proteins of influenza A did not result in an increase in incidence.

Finally, another notable vaccine technique is the epitope-based Multimeric-001 (M-001) candidate vaccine, which is now being tested in clinical trials. This vaccine, initially published by Ben-Yedidia et al. and later produced by BiondVax Pharmaceuticals Ltd., is made up of B- and T-cell epitopes taken from influenza A and B strains, containing nine conserved epitopes from the HA (including the globular head), NP, and M1 proteins [38, 52, 53]. To compensate for M-001 peptides' poor immunogenicity and expensive cost, the epitopes are concatenated in triplicate into a single recombinant protein generated in E. coli. M-001 has been evaluated in both preclinical and clinical research, and it has been shown to protect mice against infection with various influenza strains while also being safe and generating both B- and T-cell specific immune responses [38, 53]. However, M-001 alone does not elicit HAI antibodies, which can only be generated when M-001 is followed by a boosting with seasonal or pandemic strain specific vaccinations [54].

4. Conclusion

Influenza virus infection is a continuing health and economic burden that causes epidemics with pandemic potential, impacting 5–30% of the world population each year and resulting in millions of hospitalizations and thousands of fatalities. Because of its great vulnerability to antigenic variation, influenza A is the type most responsible for pandemics. Influenza is extremely infectious, with symptoms including fever, cough, chills or sweats, myalgias, and malaise. The hypervariability of the amino acid sequences encoding HA and NA is primarily responsible for epidemic and pandemic influenza epidemics, which are the result of antigenic drift or shift. As a result, research on an effective broadly-reactive influenza vaccine capable of providing protection against both seasonal and pandemic influenza is now underway.

Conflict of interest

The authors declare no conflict of interests.

Author details

Babayemi Olawale Oladejo* and Covenant Femi Adeboboye
Department of Microbiology, Federal University of Technology, Akure, Nigeria

*Address all correspondence to: booladejo@futa.edu.ng

References

[1] Jung HE, Lee HK. Host protective immune responses against influenza A virus infection. Viruses. 2020;**12**:504. DOI: 10.3390/v12050504

[2] CDC, Hall E. Influenza2021. pp. 179-192 Available from: https://www.cdc.gov/vaccines/pubs/pinkbook/flu.html

[3] Bullard BL, Weaver EA. Strategies targeting hemagglutinin as a universal influenza vaccine. Vaccine. 2021;**9**:257. DOI: 10.3390/vaccines9030257

[4] Chen X, Liu S, Goraya MU, Maarouf M, Huang S, Chen J-L. Host immune response to influenza A virus infection. Frontiers in Immunology. 2018;**9**:320. DOI: 10.3389/fimmu.2018.00320

[5] Andre CK, Paul GT. Influenza virus-related critical illness: Pathophysiology and epidemiology. Critical Care. 2019;**23**:258. DOI: 10.1186/s13054-019-2539-x

[6] World health organization (WHO). Influenza Virus Infections in Humans. WHO. Available from: http://www.who.int/influenza/gisrs_laboratory/terminology_variant/en/index.html; 2014 http://www.who.int/entity/influenza/human_animal_interface/influenza_h7n9/H7N9VirusNaming_16Apr13.pdf

[7] Susanne H, Christin B, Karen MR, Scott B. Influenza virus-induced lung injury: Pathogenesis and implications for treatment. The European Respiratory Journal. 2015;**45**:1463-1478. DOI: 10.1183/09031936.00186214

[8] Zangrillo A, Biondi-Zoccai G, Landoni G, Frati G, Patroniti N, Pesenti A, et al. Extracorporeal membrane oxygenation (ECMO) in patients with H1N1 influenza infection: A systematic review and meta-analysis including 8 studies and 266 patients receiving ECMO. Critical Care. 2013;**17**(1):R30

[9] Kadoglou NPE, Bracke F, Simmers T, Tsiodras S, Parissis J. Influenza infection and heart failure-vaccination may change heart failure prognosis? Heart Failure Reviews. 2017;**22**(3):329-336

[10] Kwong JC, Schwartz KL, Campitelli MA. Acute myocardial infarction after laboratory-confirmed influenza infection. The New England Journal of Medicine. 2018;**378**(26):2540-2541

[11] Adeboboye C, Oladejo B, Adebolu T. Immunomodulation: A broad perspective for patients' survival of COVID-19 infection. European Journal of Biological Research. 2020;**10**:217-224

[12] Huang C, Wang Y, Li X, et al. Clinical features of patients infected with 2019 novel coronavirus in Wuhan, China. Lancet. 2020;**395**(10223):497-506

[13] Xu ZL, Shi L, Wang Y, et al. Pathological findings of COVID-19 associated with acute respiratory distress syndrome. The Lancet Respiratory Medicine. 2020;**8**(4):420-422

[14] Jose JR, Manuel A. COVID-19 cytokine storm: The interplay between inflammation and coagulation. The Lancet Respiratory Medicine. 2020;**S2213-2600**(20):30216-30212

[15] Oladejo B, Adeboboye C, Adebolu T. Understanding the genetic determinant of severity in viral diseases: A case of SARS-Cov-2 infection. Egyptian Journal of Medical Human Genetics. 2020;**21**:77. DOI: 10.1186/s43042-020-00122-z

[16] Cao B, Li XW, Mao Y, et al. Clinical features of the initial cases of 2009 pandemic influenza A (H1N1) virus infection in China. The New England Journal of Medicine. 2009;**361**:2507-2517

[17] Jain S, Kamimoto L, Bramley AM, et al. Hospitalized patients with 2009 H1N1 influenza in the United States, April–June 2009. The New England Journal of Medicine. 2009;**361**:1935-1944

[18] Estenssoro E, Ríos FG, Apezteguía C, et al. Pandemic 2009 influenza A in Argentina: A study of 337 patients on mechanical ventilation. American Journal of Respiratory and Critical Care Medicine. 2010;**182**:41-48

[19] Riscili BP, Anderson TB, Prescott HC, et al. An assessment of h1n1 influenza-associated acute respiratory distress syndrome severity after adjustment for treatment characteristics. PLoS ONE. 2011;**6**:e18166

[20] Kuiken T, Taubenberger J. Pathology of human influenza revisited. Vaccine. 2008;**26**:D59-D66

[21] Short KR, Kroeze EJ, Fouchier RA, et al. Pathogenesis of influenza-induced acute respiratory distress syndrome. The Lancet Infectious Diseases. 2014;**14**:57-69

[22] Bautista E, Chotpitayasunondh T, Gao Z, et al. Clinical aspects of pandemic 2009 influenza A (H1N1) virus infection. The New England Journal of Medicine. 2010;**362**:1708-1719

[23] David Y, Gaitonde MD, Faith C, Moore MC, Mackenzie KM. (Dwight D. Eisenhower, Army Medical Center, Fort Gordon, Georgia)Influenza: Diagnosis and Treatment. American Family Physician. Available from: www.aafp.org/afp; 2019

[24] Centers for Disease Control and Prevention. Influenza (flu): for clinicians: antiviral medication. 2018. Accessed: February 2, 2022. Available from: https://www.cdc.gov/flu/professionals/antivirals/summary-clinicians.htm

[25] Schmitz N, Kurrer M, Bachmann M, Kopf M. Interleukin-1 is responsible for acute lung immunopathology but increases survival of respiratory influenza virus infection. Journal of Virology. 2005;**79**(10):6441-6448. DOI: 10.1128/JVI.79.10.6441-6448.2005

[26] Beigel J, Bray M. Current and future antiviral therapy of severe seasonal and avian influenza. Antiviral Research. 2008;**78**(1):91-102. DOI: 10.1016/j.antiviral.2008.01.003

[27] Ferguson NM, Cummings DA, Cauchemez S, Fraser C, Riley S, Meeyai A, et al. Strategies for containing an emerging influenza pandemic in Southeast Asia. Nature. 2005;**437**(7056):209-214. DOI: 10.1038/nature04017

[28] Carrat F, Vergu E, Ferguson NM, Lemaitre M, Cauchemez S, Leach S, et al. Time lines of infection and disease in human influenza: A review of volunteer challenge studies. American Journal of Epidemiology. 2008;**167**(7):775-785. DOI: 10.1093/aje/kwm375

[29] Davies WL, Hoffmann CE, Paulshock M, Wood TR, Haff RF, Grunert RR, et al. Antiviral activity of 1-adamantanamine (amantadine). Science. 1964;**144**:862-863. DOI: 10.1126/science.144.3620.862

[30] Lv HM, Guo XL, Gu RX, Wei DQ. Free energy calculations and binding analysis of two potential anti-influenza drugs with polymerase basic protein-2 (PB2). Protein and Peptide Letters. 2011;**18**:1002-1009. DOI: 10.2174/092986611796378675

[31] Schmidtke M, Schnittler U, Jahn B, Dahse HM, Stelzner A. A rapid assay for evaluation of antiviral activity against coxsackie virus B3, influenza virus a, and herpes simplex virus type 1. Journal of Virological Methods. 2001;**95**:133-143. DOI: 10.1016/s0166-0934(01)00305-6

[32] Hung HC, Liu CL, Hsu JTA, Horng JT, Fang MY, Wu SY, et al. Development of an anti-influenza drug screening assay targeting nucleoproteins with tryptophan fluorescence quenching. Analytical Chemistry. 2012;**84**:6391-6399. DOI: 10.1021/ac2022426

[33] Dai JP, Wang GF, Li WZ, Zhang L, Yang JC, Zhao XF, et al. High-throughput screening for anti-influenza A virus drugs and study of the mechanism of procyanidin on influenza A virus induced autophagy. Journal of Biomolecular Screening. 2012;**17**:605-617. DOI: 10.1177/1087057111435236

[34] Yamada K, Koyama H, Hagiwara K, Ueda A, Sasaki Y, Kanesashi S, et al. Identification of a novel compound with antiviral activity against influenza A virus depending on PA subunit of viral RNA polymerase. Microbes and Infection. 2012;**14**:740-747. DOI: 10.1016/j.micinf.2012.02.012

[35] Sauerbrei A, Haertl A, Brandstaedt A, Schmidtke M, Wutzler P. Utilization of the embryonated egg for in vivo evaluation of the anti-influenza virus activity of neuraminidase inhibitors. Medical Microbiology and Immunology. 2006;**195**:65-71. DOI: 10.1007/s00430-005-0002-x

[36] Cao B, Wang DY, Yu XM, We LQ, Pu ZH, Gao Y, et al. An uncontrolled open label, multicenter study to monitor the antiviral activity and safety of inhaled zanamivir (as Rotadisk via Diskhaler device) among Chinese adolescents and adults with influenza-like illness. Chinese Medical Journal. 2012;**125**:3002-3007. DOI: 10.3760/cma.j.issn.0366-6999.2012.17.007

[37] Gutierrez-Pizarraya A, Perez-Romero P, Alvarez R, Aydillo TA, Osorio-Gomez G, Milara-Ibanez C, et al. Unexpected severity of cases of influenza B infection in patients that required hospitalization during the first post-pandemic wave. The Journal of Infection. 2012;**65**:423-430

[38] Sautto GA, Kirchenbaum GA, Ross TM. Towards a universal influenza vaccine: Different approaches for one goal. Virology Journal. 2018;**15**:17

[39] Chambers BS, Parkhouse K, Ross TM, Alby K, Hensley SE. Identification of hemagglutinin residues responsible for H3N2 antigenic drift during the 2014-2015 influenza season. Cell Reports. 2015;**12**:1-6

[40] Nachbagauer R, Liu W-C, Choi A, Wohlbold TJ, Atlas T, Rajendran M, et al. A universal influenza virus vaccine candidate confers protection against pandemic H1N1 infection in preclinical ferret studies. Vaccine. 2017;**2**:26

[41] Nachbagauer R, Palese P. Is a Universal Influenza Virus Vaccine Possible? Annual Review of Medicine. 2020;**71**(18):1-18. 13. DOI: 10.1146/annurev-med-120617-041310

[42] Impagliazzo A, Milder F, Kuipers H, Wagner MV, Zhu X, Hoffman RM, et al. A stable trimeric influenza hemagglutinin stem as a broadly protective immunogen. Science. 2015;**349**:1301-1306

[43] Mancini N, Solforosi L, Clementi N, De Marco D, Clementi M, Burioni R. A potential role for monoclonal antibodies in prophylactic and therapeutic

treatment of influenza. Antiviral Research. 2011;**92**:15-26

[44] Giles BM, Ross TM. A computationally optimized broadly reactive antigen (COBRA) based H5N1 VLP vaccine elicits broadly reactive antibodies in mice and ferrets. Vaccine. 2011;**29**:3043-3054

[45] Wong TM, Ross TM. Use of computational and recombinant technologies for developing novel influenza vaccines. Expert Review of Vaccines. 2016;**15**:41-51

[46] Carter DM, Darby CA, Lefoley BC, Crevar CJ, Alefantis T, Oomen R, et al. Design and characterization of a computationally optimized broadly reactive hemagglutinin vaccine for H1N1 influenza viruses. Journal of Virology. 2016;**90**:4720-4734

[47] Strauch EM, Bernard SM, La D, Bohn AJ, Lee PS, Anderson CE, et al. Computational design of trimeric influenza-neutralizing proteins targeting the hemagglutinin receptor binding site. Nature Biotechnology. 2017;**35**:667-671

[48] Wong TM, Allen JD, Bebin-Blackwell AG, Carter DM, Alefantis T, DiNapoli J, et al. COBRA HA elicits hemagglutination-inhibition antibodies against a panel of H3N2 influenza virus co-circulating variants. Journal of Virology. 2017;**91**(24):e01581-e01517. DOI: 10.1128/JVI.01581-17

[49] Giles BM, Crevar CJ, Carter DM, Bissel SJ, Schultz-Cherry S, Wiley CA, et al. A computationally optimized hemagglutinin virus-like particle vaccine elicits broadly reactive antibodies that protect nonhuman primates from H5N1 infection. The Journal of Infectious Diseases. 2012;**205**:1562-1570

[50] Song L, Xiong D, Kang X, Yang Y, Wang J, Guo Y, et al. An avian influenza A (H7N9) virus vaccine candidate based on the fusion protein of hemagglutinin globular head and salmonella typhimurium flagellin. BMC Biotechnology. 2015;**15**:79

[51] Evans TG, Bussey L, Eagling-Vose E, Rutkowski K, Ellis C, Argent C, et al. Efficacy and safety of a universal influenza A vaccine (MVA-NP+M1) in adults when given after seasonal quadrivalent influenza vaccine immunisation (FLU009): A phase 2b, randomised, double-blind trial. The Lancet Infectious Diseases. 2022;**21**:1473-3099. DOI: 10.1016/S1473-3099(21)00702-7

[52] Ben-Yedidia T, Marcus H, Reisner Y, Arnon R. Intranasal administration of peptide vaccine protects human/mouse radiation chimera from influenza infection. International Immunology. 1999;**11**:1043-1051

[53] Adar Y, Singer Y, Levi R, Tzehoval E, Perk S, Banet-Noach C, et al. A universal epitope-based influenza vaccine and its efficacy against H5N1. Vaccine. 2009;**27**:2099-2107

[54] Atsmon J, Caraco Y, Ziv-Sefer S, Shaikevich D, Abramov E, Volokhov I, et al. Priming by a novel universal influenza vaccine (Multimeric-001)-a gateway for improving immune response in the elderly population. Vaccine. 2014;**32**:5816-5823

Section 3

COVID-19

Chapter 4

COVID-19 Prevention through Vitamin C, D, and Zinc Supplementation: A Small Clinical Study in Two Parts

Chanda Siddoo-Atwal

Abstract

At the time of this study India had the third highest COVID-19 infection rate in the world after the US and Brazil, but that statistic was in flux due to rapidly changing variables and, therefore, it seemed an appropriate setting for a supplementation study. Following a successful first trial of vitamin C, D and zinc supplementation in 2020 with the staff at a small medical clinic in India, a second opportunity arose to continue the trial from January-March 22nd due to an urban coronavirus outbreak during the beginning of March 2021. It resulted in nearly a doubling of COVID-19 cases within the country in two weeks (March 8th - March 22nd) possibly due to the new, highly infectious, Indian Delta variant with multiple mutations and/or other international variants like the UK Alpha variant that were also present in the population by this time. As a result, a nighttime curfew and other restrictions were imposed for the whole month. An outbreak also occurred locally in a nearby city where the incidence of coronavirus cases increased and this happened prior to vaccination of the medical staff as part of the country's universal inoculation campaign for healthcare workers, which began in January 2021 (one clinic clerk who travelled to the district civil hospital to receive the vaccine during the course of this second study was disqualified; all other clinic staff were inoculated after March 22nd). Although the clinic had closed during the first lockdown between March and mid-June 2020, it remained open to the public for this second wave in March 2021. During this period, the medical & non-medical staff continued following the same supplementation regimen as they had in July-December 2020 for Part I of this trial with positive results. Once again, in Part II of the trial, there were no COVID-19 cases recorded among any of the staff members at the clinic, which is situated in a rural community. It was concluded that targeted vitamin/mineral supplementation may be a useful addition to the anti-COVID-19 arsenal for health professionals at higher than average risk of infection.

Keywords: novel coronavirus, SARS-CoV-2, COVID-19, vitamin C, vitamin D, zinc

1. Introduction

A baffling number of disparate symptoms have been ascribed to COVID-19 infection including respiratory, gastrointestinal, circulatory, urinary tract and nerve dysfunction that has resulted in multi-organ failure in some cases. An array of risk factors has also been identified ranging from age, sex, obesity, diabetes, and hypertension to cigarette smoking that can increase mortality rate dramatically [1]. So far, a surprising number of deaths have been recorded worldwide due to the coronavirus pandemic and the figure has surpassed the 5.5 million mark [2].

1.1 Symptoms

In general, COVID-19 infection is associated with the increased production of pro-inflammatory cytokines, C-reactive protein, increased risk of pneumonia, sepsis, acute respiratory distress syndrome, and heart failure [3]. Early reports from China suggested the most common symptoms of COVID-19 infection were fever (88%) and dry cough (67.7%). Rhinorrhea (4.9%) and gastrointestinal symptoms (diarrhea 4–14%) were less common [4].

It has been concluded that COVID-19 may predispose to both venous and arterial thromboembolism due to excessive inflammation, hypoxia, immobilization, and diffuse intravascular coagulation [5]. In addition, the COVID-19 pandemic is associated with neurological symptoms and complications including anosmia, hypogeusia, seizures, and stroke [6]. COVID-19 complications in the brain can include delirium, inflammation, and encephalitis [7]. A temporary loss of smell (anosmia) can be a consistent indicator of COVID-19 infection [8]. COVID-19 is now recognized as a multi-organ disease with a broad range of effects. An unusually long recovery period also seems to be a common aftermath of COVID-19 (post-acute COVID-19 syndrome or, popularly, long-COVID) and may involve one or more of various clinical manifestations including fatigue/muscular weakness, joint pain, dyspnea, cough, sleep and cognitive disturbances, headaches, anxiety/depression, palpitations, chest pain, thromboembolism, chronic kidney disease, and hair loss [9].

Even though, initially, children were thought to be unaffected by the novel coronavirus, a cluster of children with hyperinflammatory shock and features similar to Kawasaki disease and toxic shock syndrome was first reported in England. Almost all these pediatric cases had positive SARS-CoV-2 test results. This hyperinflammatory condition can include serious inflammation of the blood vessels and coronary arteries. Consequently, this illness has been termed COVID-19-associated multisystem inflammatory syndrome [10].

1.2 Internal risk factors

Some scientists have opined that COVID-19 is highly contagious and highly lethal to a small subset of the population, while it produces milder symptoms in most people. Although, the SARS-CoV-2 virus infects people of all ages, the World Health Organization (WHO) has determined that the evidence to date suggests that older adults and adults with underlying medical conditions are at a higher risk of developing severe COVID-19 disease [11]. However, recent new mutations in variants of the virus may be shifting the age demographic to include younger populations under the age of 60 as reflected in the sudden rise in fatalities among young and middle-aged adults after identification of the Brazilian Gamma variant [12].

One large study seems to indicate that obesity, high blood pressure, and diabetes are strong risk factors for COVID-19 [13]. It has also been observed that cardiovascular disease and respiratory diseases could greatly affect the prognosis [14]. In fact, in an interesting study involving autopsies on 12 COVID-19 patients, the results revealed that coronary heart disease and asthma were common comorbid conditions in 50% of the deceased [15]. Other research suggests that certain cancer patients are more vulnerable to COVID-19 infection [16]. In addition, a surprising gender disparity appears to be present about SARS-CoV-2 infection. Statistics from Australia, Belgium, Germany, Italy, the Netherlands, South Korea, Spain, the UK and the US reveal that mortality rates from the virus are significantly higher in infected males than in infected females [17]. In the largest Chinese study to date assessing the severity of coronavirus infection in smokers, it was found that higher percentages of current and former smokers needed ICU support or mechanical ventilation. Higher percentages of smokers among the severe cases also died [18].

1.3 External risk factors

Italian researchers have proposed an association between higher mortality rates in Northern Italy and peaks of particulate matter concentrations in this region. The most polluted northern provinces of Italy were found to have more infection cases than the less polluted southern provinces and this correlated well with ambient particulate matter concentrations that often exceeded the legal limit in these areas [19].

This could have been a significant factor in the spread of the coronavirus in highly polluted and populated cities like Mumbai, India. Social conditions such as crowding in slums have also been considered contributory to the dispersal of the virus in developing countries like Brazil and India. Proximity to infected individuals increases the risk of person-to-person transmission since the SARS-CoV-2 virus is spread mainly by respiratory droplets, but can be aerosolized, as well [20].

No matter how healthy an individual may be, the more exposure they have to a particular virus, the greater risk they have of contracting the disease. The greater the number of particles of the virus one is exposed to, the greater the chance that they will overwhelm the body and immune responses. This is the reason that frontline healthcare workers have been getting serious cases of COVID-19 and, particularly, middle-aged male general practitioners have been dying at a higher frequency than the general population [21, 22].

1.4 Rise of the coronavirus variants

According to available information, during the first part of this study initiated in July 2020, the original strain of the novel coronavirus from Wuhan, China was the main agent of infection in India due to business travel, tourism, and trade between the two neighboring nations before lockdown and no vaccines were available [1]. In China, this would extend in the form of a ban on non-resident travelers from March 2020 and lifting it would not be contemplated until the February 2022 Winter Olympics.

Subsequently, the Alpha coronavirus variant, which had spread at least 50% faster than earlier lineages was linked to a rise in cases in southeast England by public health officials in November 2020. Approximately around the same time, the Beta variant was detected in South Africa and linked to the second wave of infections in the country. Not long after, the highly transmissible Gamma variant was localized to Amazonas state in Brazil. These three variants shared some common mutations, particularly in key regions of the spike protein that is involved in recognizing the host-cell ACE2 receptors used by the virus for entering human cells [1, 23].

Thus, by the time the second part of this study was undertaken in January 2021, the Alpha, Beta, and Gamma variants were also present within the Indian population and the UK variant became the dominant strain in Punjab state mainly due to unimpeded travel abroad [24]. Simultaneously, the homegrown Delta variant with multiple mutations had become dominant in the Indian state of Maharashtra and several factors such as large public gatherings at celebrations like Holi, which were not tightly restricted, are likely to have contributed to the precipitous rise of Delta within the country. Moreover, people had started to mingle socially without restraint and to travel to adjoining states thereby distributing the virus and its variants, notably Delta [24]. This is probably what lead to nearly a doubling of cases in March [23]. Up to this point, vaccines had not been available, but became available to the clinic staff shortly after in April, 2021. Soon, the Delta variant had been exported all over India, back to China, and around the world, where it became the predominant strain in many places due to its high transmissibility [24, 25].

2. Methods

Just until recently, India has had the second or third highest COVID-19 infection rate in the world. However, the mortality rate has been comparatively low, possibly due to a relatively younger average age of the general population. There is another current hypothesis that a national Bacillus Calmette-Guérin (BCG) vaccination program in countries seems to be associated with reduced mortality from COVID-19 and India has such a program [26]. This purely observational study to establish dosage and tolerance of prolonged vitamin and mineral supplementation was carried out at a private clinic located in a small town in the District of Nawan Shahr near the historic city of Rahon in North India (Kapoor Singh Canadian Hospital). There were 7500 inhabitants in the town and a total of five COVID-19 cases (4 male and 1 female) between March (when the epidemic began in India) and December 2020. Interestingly, there were no mortalities among these patients who were quarantined in a neighboring city and one of the main treatments current in India at this time was the malarial medication, chloroquine, which also displays anti-inflammatory activity [27]. There was a total state-wide lockdown between March and mid-June 2020. The clinic decided to re-open in July 2020 following the lockdown in the absence of any available coronavirus vaccine. During the second part of the study (January–March 22, 2021), approximately 50 coronavirus cases were recorded in this small town & adjoining village with a total of 1 or 2 deaths as a result of COVID-19 infection. At this stage, treatment at civil hospitals included steroids and antibiotics such as azithromycin for secondary infections [28]. Testing was also more widely available during this second surge, which started in March, peaked in May, and started to subside in October 2021.

The clinic that took part in this trial employed a total of 15 staff members; 9 men and 6 women. They included 2 doctors (one male, one female), 3 nurses, 2 laboratory technicians, 1 security guard, 1 cleaner and 6 general maintenance staff. All participants consented to take part in the study. Although, all 15 staff members participated in the first part of the study, one general staff member (a clinic clerk) dropped out of the second part of the study as a result of being vaccinated and thereby reduced the test group to 14. Although, the medical staff (7) were aware of the potential benefits of supplementation, the non-medical staff members (7/8) were not aware of the potential health benefits. However, they were informed that the supplements were not harmful in any way. In addition, all the non-medical staff was not equally exposed to patients as the medical staff. Each staff member took part voluntarily in the first trial that was initiated on July 1, 2020 and extended to December 31, 2020 and in the second trial that was initiated on January 1 and extended to March 22, 2021. It is unlikely that the townspeople were taking oral dietary supplements of any kind since they are not that popular in India and provided the background population for this study. The background population establishes the presence of active coronavirus cases in the community and forms a basis for comparison.

Vitamin, mineral, and amino acid supplementation is not an uncommon practice at European health clinics. For example, specific combinations of vitamins and minerals may be used to promote general good health. One such formula prescribed at a German vegetarian health clinic (Schlosspark Klink) included CoQ-10 (which stimulates ATP production), vitamin D3, and zinc. Supplementary protein pills were used regularly to complement the diet and boost the body's overall metabolism in patients. Moreover, during the SARS-CoV-2 pandemic, they routinely recommended 20,000 IU per week of vitamin D3 (spring to fall) and 40,000 IU per week of vitamin D3 (winter months) as a preventive measure to their guests based on laboratory blood tests, even to those who regularly included meat and fish in their diet. Vitamin D was measured in blood samples from patients as *25-hydroxycholecalciferol* and a minimum concentration of 55 *ng/ml* was recommended by the clinic doctors (whereas the sufficiency scale range is 20–70 ng/ml); although anything below this value was not deemed as representing a deficiency, it was judged as being too low for effective COVID-19 prevention.

Thus, in addition to standard precautionary measures adopted universally during the pandemic, a careful selection of vitamin and mineral supplements was made to help protect the staff at the Indian clinic participating in this particular study from coronavirus infection. The supplements selected for the staff included a combined daily dose of vitamin C (500 mg) and zinc (20 mg) in tablet form [Indian Drugs & Pharmaceutical Co.] plus a weekly dose of vitamin D3 (60,000 IU) capsules [Dr Morpen; Cipla; or, Cadila Co.]. The corresponding daily dose of vitamin D3, which is significantly higher than that normally recommended in Germany (800 IU per day) and in other countries around the world such as the US (2000 IU per day), is commonly prescribed as a therapeutic dose in India possibly due to the popularity of vegetarianism. The reason for this choice of combined supplements above biological doses was as follows:

2.1 Vitamin D

Vitamin D3 (25-hydroxycholecalciferol) is the most bioavailable form of vitamin D for the human body and the bioactive form (1,25-dihydroxycholecalciferol) is synthesized by its enzymatic hydroxylation mainly in the kidney. This bioactive form of vitamin D also functions as a hormone that regulates calcium and phosphorus metabolism via a nuclear receptor that can alter the expression of genes in the intestine, kidney, and bone [29].

Vitamin D enhances cellular innate immunity partly through the induction of antimicrobial peptides, including human cathelicidin, and, defensins. Cathelicidins exhibit direct antimicrobial activities against a spectrum of microbes including many types of bacteria, enveloped and nonenveloped viruses, and fungi. The main action of these host-derived peptides is to kill the invading pathogens by perturbing their cell membranes. Moreover, it is effective in reducing concentrations of pro-inflammatory cytokines that produce the inflammation that injures the lining of the lungs leading to pneumonia during viral infections like COVID-19 and increasing concentrations of anti-inflammatory cytokines [3].

Vitamin D deficiency is a worldwide problem, but is particularly pronounced in the elderly, who are at the greatest risk of contracting severe COVID-19 infection. The release of pro-inflammatory cytokines is one of the major causative factors in serious COVID-19 infections. However, vitamin D modulates its presence in the body by preventing macrophages from releasing too many inflammatory cytokines and chemokines. Calcitriol has also been found to exert an influence on ACE-2 receptors. Thus, it is not surprising that vitamin D deficiency has been correlated with COVID-19 cases and an increased risk of mortality in a European study [30]. Conversely, medical doctors in Eastern Europe have rarely found COVID-19 patients with vitamin D sufficiency to require ICU stays in hospital (personal communication from Dr. Martin von Rosen, MD).

2.2 Zinc

RNA synthesis occurs in the life cycle of the SARS-CoV-1 virus to reproduce its genetic material and is catalyzed by an RNA-dependent RNA polymerase, which is the core enzyme of a multiprotein replication/transcription complex. In the case of SARS-CoV-1, an excess of intracellular zinc ions has been found to efficiently inhibit the RNA-synthesizing activity of this replication and transcription multiprotein. Enzymatic studies in vitro have revealed that zinc directly blocks the activity of the RNA polymerase by inhibiting elongation and reducing template binding. This RNA polymerase core, which is a central component of the coronaviral replication/transcription machinery, is well conserved among the members of the coronavirus family including SARS-CoV-2 [31, 32]. Therefore, it is quite possible that zinc treatment would have a similar biochemical effect on SARS-CoV-2 and interfere with its ability to replicate.

In the human body, zinc displays antiviral effects by modulating the type I Interferon response and performs a variety of vital antioxidant functions [33]. Inside the cell, the harmful effects of free radicals are balanced by the action of antioxidant enzymes (such as copper-zinc superoxide dismutase) and non-enzymatic antioxidants (such as metallothioneins), which utilize zinc and help to regulate its intracellular levels [34, 35]. There are several other ways zinc functions in both adaptive and innate immune systems, as well. It regulates the proliferation, differentiation, maturation and functioning of lymphocytes, and other leukocytes. In addition, zinc regulates the immune response, and its deficiency increases susceptibility to inflammatory and infectious diseases, including pneumonia. Moreover, zinc deficiency may be present in 17% of the world's population [36]. Interestingly, a trial with four COVID-19 patients suggested that therapy with high dose zinc salt oral lozenges [up to 200 mg/day] initiated a significant reduction of disease symptoms within 24 hours [37]. Short-term zinc use at these doses is considered safe [38]. Thus, low-risk ways of increasing zinc bioavailability in the body above biological levels can be safely considered.

2.3 Vitamin C

Vitamin C is known as an essential anti-oxidant that efficiently quenches damaging free radicals produced during normal metabolic respiration by the body and it functions as an enzymatic co-factor for physiological reactions such as hormone production, collagen synthesis and immune potentiation [39]. In addition, the anti-inflammatory action of ascorbic acid is evidenced in several cytoprotective functions under physiological conditions, including the prevention of DNA mutation induced by oxidation. In fact, it has been established in *in vivo* studies that the consumption of vitamin C-rich foods is inversely correlated with the level of oxidative DNA damage [40]. Moreover, vitamin C is a well-known anti-viral agent that has been demonstrated to show anti-viral immune responses, especially against the influenza virus at the onset of infection by the increased production of IFN-α/β [39]. There has also been some interesting evidence that oral vitamin C (2–8 g/day) may reduce the incidence and duration of respiratory infections, while intravenous vitamin C has been shown to reduce mortality, ICU and hospital stays, and time on mechanical ventilation in severe respiratory infections. Vitamin C deficiency has been observed in many respiratory infections, as well, and a recent study from New Zealand reported that patients with pneumonia had depleted vitamin C levels as compared with healthy controls suggesting that it may be potentially helpful in the treatment of COVID-19 at therapeutic doses [41].

3. Results

On average, the clinic was visited by 60 patients per day during July–December, 2020 and 45 patients per day during January–March 22, 2021. Thermal scanning was instituted at the clinic gates and any patient with a fever was seated outside and given a week's supply of vitamin C plus zinc tablets, vitamin D capsules, and aspirin. The patients without fever were allowed inside the clinic compound after receiving hand sanitizer and a disposable mask. They were instructed to keep a 2-meter distance between themselves and other patients as they waited on chairs outside the clinic. Only 6 patients were allowed into the clinic waiting room at one time (while 10–12 is the usual number). All patients with cold symptoms other than fever also received oral vitamin C/zinc and vitamin D3 supplements. All the hospital staff wore medical masks. PPE was not considered necessary as there were relatively few coronavirus cases locally and anyone with a higher than the normal temperature was not allowed inside the clinic. So, the hazard was not deemed to be extreme. Infected individuals in the district were immediately removed to pre-designated quarantine locations by government health inspectors where they received medical treatment for 2 weeks.

There were no adverse reactions to the special selective supplementation in any of the staff members during the first or second trial. There were no COVID-19 cases recorded among any of the staff members for the duration of this preliminary study, even though, approximately a third of them were living in and commuting from nearby towns and cities where the incidence rate was higher. The length of this trial suggests that there was ample opportunity for COVID-19 infection to occur in any of the subjects, especially since routine social distancing was not being observed during much of this time in India. All the subjects would have been exposed to potential virus carriers during work hours at the clinic (via asymptomatic carriers or those with cold symptoms other than fever), on public transport, and at home in their social circle. Similarly, the townspeople often traveled on public transport to other towns and cities and would have been exposed to potentially infected individuals at social gatherings.

4. Discussion

Although, there is much interest in vitamin C, D, and zinc in the coronavirus literature, currently there is scant data about the potential synergistic role of these three supplements in COVID-19 prevention and clinical studies are lacking. Clinical trials for treating COVID-19 patients with these supplements are slightly more common; however, they usually do not focus on all three supplements together. Thus, the clinical study presented here appears to be the first of its kind [42].

A small two-part clinical trial with 14–15 subjects was undertaken to test the feasibility of taking specific supplements with anti-viral properties to aid in the prevention of COVID-19 infection, namely, vitamin C (500 mg/day), vitamin D (60,0000 IU/week), and zinc (20 mg/day) before the availability of any vaccine. It was concluded that this type of targeted supplementation of medical professionals and healthcare workers in an environment of potentially heightened exposure to coronavirus could be beneficial at the established dosages, which were non-biological doses well above corresponding biological doses. The combination of vitamins and mineral included in this preliminary study was selected for its special qualities in potentially combatting the coronavirus and was well-tolerated. On a biochemical level, the vitamin C likely acted by increasing the production of anti-viral Interferon α/β; vitamin D stimulated the secretion of antimicrobial peptides (defensins and cathelicidins) which perturb microbe cell membranes; and, zinc boosted the immune response in the subjects to ward off infection. Zinc may also have provided a secondary defense to clinic staff members by interfering with the SARS-CoV-2 replication machinery and disabling the viral RNA polymerase of invading virus particles. No other supplements aside from these three were provided to the participants to minimize confounding variables.

Even though, a variety of vaccines did become available following this study and all the clinic staff opted to be fully vaccinated (the vaccine supplied to healthcare workers in India was mainly Covishield), it was decided to continue with this special supplementation regimen (the vitamin D3 dose was gradually reduced to 30,000 IU per week), even after the six-month and two-and-three quarter month trial periods for several reasons. Firstly, it is not known, yet, exactly how long the antibody immunity generated by these vaccines lasts (although an estimate of 3–6 months has been suggested) and, therefore, there may be a lag period during which recipients are not protected. Lasting immunity following acute viral infection is variable and pathogen-specific ranging from life-long for smallpox or measles, to highly transient for common cold coronaviruses (CCC). It often requires maintenance of both serum antibody and antigen-specific memory B and T lymphocytes. Secondly, as new variant strains of the novel coronavirus continue to appear and change beyond recognition, many of the vaccines may become less effective or even ineffective at some point as antibodies can no longer recognize their corresponding antigens. For example, the Alpha, Beta, and Delta coronavirus mutant strains appear to have a modified spike protein with an increased binding capacity. The Gamma variant carries some of the same spike mutations [23]. This feature may render vaccines that target solely the novel coronavirus spike protein irrelevant. Evidence is already emerging that suggests fast-spreading coronavirus variants like Omicron with an ever-increasing number of multiple mutations in the spike protein may evade the main immune responses triggered by many vaccines and natural infection [43–47] possibly excluding T cell immunity [48, 49]. Thus, it is preferrable to seek protection simultaneously from several biochemical sources that disable different parts of the viral machinery. Thirdly, even though it is possible to alter existing vaccines to target these new variants, it takes some time to re-engineer them, so it is not desirable for recipients to have an unprotected interval. Finally, there is the question of how many vaccines an individual can safely receive each year without engendering negative physiological consequences or increasing the chances of experiencing long-term side-effects.

As an example, *thimerosal* is a mercury-containing organic compound (approximately 50% mercury by weight) that has been widely used as a preservative in many inactivated-virus vaccines since the 1930s [50]. Mercury is toxic to both animals and humans and is associated with several adverse health effects including anemia, cardiovascular disease, developmental abnormalities, neurobehavioral disorders, kidney and liver damage, and brain cancer [51]. Although, it is claimed that thimerosal is safe in small doses, it is unlikely that experiments have been conducted on human subjects receiving two to three or more vaccines per year as seems to be required in the case of coronavirus. Not all the new coronavirus vaccines like the mRNA vaccines contain thimerosal, but there may be other ingredients with unintended future consequences, which have not been adequately tested. Naturally, these could have the greatest negative impact on younger members of the population. Therefore, the most prudent approach for government health agencies to adopt may be to continue to offer annual booster vaccines for those 60 years or over and to other vulnerable members of society.

Further issues with the various available vaccines have also come to light. For example, in rare instances, the AstraZeneca COVID-19 vaccine has been linked to blood clots, while the Pfizer and Moderna vaccines have been associated with severe allergic reactions in rare cases [52, 53]. It may be possible to mitigate some of these ill-effects by adjusting the vaccine dose according to a recipient's weight (for example, a person who weighs 45 kg might receive a lesser dose than someone who weighs 90 kg or double their weight). Moreover, COVID-19 vaccination is associated with a lower risk of several, but not necessarily all, COVID-19 symptoms in those with breakthrough SARS-CoV-2 infection including long-COVID features, renal disease, mood, anxiety, and sleep disorders [54]. However, there were no breakthrough cases of COVID-19 between April and December 2021 in any of the 14 hospital staff members who had been vaccinated, but simultaneously continued with supplementation. No mild cold-like symptoms were observed in any of the subjects either. It is also worth noting that none of the staff received a booster vaccine during this period, which would only become available to healthcare workers and medical professionals in January 2022. Thus, this study successfully spanned the rise of Alpha to Delta variants (*pre-vaccine*), while breakthrough cases were averted during the peak and decline of Delta and the onset of Omicron in India (*post-vaccine*).

Unfortunately, the small sample size (14, 15) of the test group in these trials could not be analyzed statistically in relation to the much larger population in the town, which merely formed a general basis for comparison. So, this may be regarded as an uncontrolled study without matched controls. Ideally, another private clinic of similar size with equivalent numbers of medical and non-medical staff members, who were not receiving supplementation, could have participated as the control group. A second similar placebo group might also have been informative. However, this would not be possible in any future studies as vaccines have become widely available to healthcare workers all over the country. At the same time, it is likely that the other hygienic practices adopted at the clinic during the pandemic may have contributed to the positive result. Moreover, the annual incidence of coronavirus cases was relatively low in the town as compared with urban centres and must also be taken into consideration. Nevertheless, it is more than likely that the clinic staff were exposed to persons infected with the coronavirus during the study (initially, the original strain, followed by the Alpha variant, at least, according to the region, and, then, later, the Delta variant), but local sequencing data was not available. Therefore, some interesting insights into supplementation with specific vitamins and minerals of medical personnel may have been gained as a result of these initial findings as no COVID-19 infections occurred among the *unvaccinated* hospital staff between July 1, 2020 and March 22, 2021 (**Tables 1** and **2**). No breakthrough infections occurred either in the staff members, who were *fully vaccinated* with the Covishield vaccine, between April and December 2021 with continued supplementation (**Table 3**). These results may prove useful for further clinical research into COVID-19 prevention, but, due to the small sample size, future studies should be conducted with much larger test groups, equally matched controls, placebo groups, and a complete statistical analysis. It may be particularly relevant for lower-income countries without immediate access to vaccines always and as an added precaution for healthcare professionals at higher-than-average risk of infection. This is also especially applicable in the event of waning vaccine efficacy as may be the case with the Omicron variant and some of its sub-variants, which seem equipped to evade antibody immunity (not necessarily T cell immunity), cause breakthrough infections, and initiate reinfections [55].

Participant's position	Daily supplement [vitamin C/Zn] (500 mg/20 mg)	Weekly supplement [vitamin D] (60,000 IU)	Coronavirus incidence (among 15 subjects)
2 doctors	+	+	−
3 nurses	+	+	−
2 lab techs	+	+	−
1 security guard	+	+	−
1 cleaning staff	+	+	−
6 general staff	+	+	−

Table 1.
Oral supplementation of staff members—Part I; pre-vaccine (July 1–December 31, 2020).

Participant's position	Daily supplement [vitamin C/Zn] (500 mg/20 mg)	Weekly supplement [vitamin D] (60,000 IU)	Coronavirus incidence (among 14 subjects)
2 doctors	+	+	−
3 nurses	+	+	−
2 lab techs	+	+	−
1 security guard	+	+	−
1 cleaning staff	+	+	−
5 general staff	+	+	−

Table 2.
Oral supplementation of staff members—Part II; pre-vaccine (January 1–March 22, 2021).

Participant's position	Daily supplement [vitamin C/Zn] (500 mg/20 mg)	Weekly supplement [vitamin D] (30–60,000 IU)	Coronavirus incidence (among 14 subjects)
2 doctors	+	+	–
3 nurses	+	+	–
2 lab techs	+	+	–
1 security guard	+	+	–
1 cleaning staff	+	+	–
5 general staff	+	+	–

Table 3.
Oral supplementation of staff members—post-vaccine (April 1–December 31, 2021).

Finally, there is no doubt that there will be ever new SARS-CoV-2 variants in the future, which may be less virulent, or possibly more so. As the virus evolves, these variants may become more transmissible and even better able to evade vaccine and natural immunity. These currently unknown mutants are beyond the scope of this book or chapter. However, the approach remains the same and we must be prepared with an artillery of weapons against the novel coronavirus rather than just relying on one.

Author details

Chanda Siddoo-Atwal[1,2,3,4]

1 University College London, England

2 Simon Fraser University, Canada

3 Medical College Wisconsin, United States

4 President and Primary Biochemist of Moondust Cosmetics Ltd., Canada

*Address all correspondence to: moondustcosmetics@gmail.com

References

[1] Siddoo-Atwal C. Chapter 2—Assembling an anti-COVID-19 artillery in the battle against the new coronavirus. In: Shah Y, Abuelzein E, editors. Some RNA Viruses. 2020. London, United Kingdom: IntechOpen; 2021. pp. 9-25. DOI: 10.5772/intechopen.95100

[2] Adam D. The pandemic's true death toll: Millions more than official counts. Nature. 2022;**601**:312-315. DOI: 10.1038/d41586-022-00104-8

[3] Grant WB, Lahore H, McDonnell SL, Baggerly CA, French CB, Aliano JL, et al. Evidence that vitamin D supplementation could reduce risk of influenza and COVID-19 infections and deaths. Nutrients. 2020;**12**(4):988. DOI: 10.3390/nu12040988

[4] He F, Deng Y, Li W. Coronavirus disease 2019: What we know? Journal of Medical Virology. 2020;**92**(7):719-725. DOI: 10.1002/jmv.25766

[5] Klok FA, Kruip MJHA, Van Der Meer NJM, Arbous MS, Gommers DAMPJ, Kant KM, et al. Incidence of thrombotic complications in critically ill ICU patients with COVID-19. Thrombosis Research. 2020;**191**(2020):145-147. DOI: 10.1016/j.thromres.2020.04.013

[6] Hess DC, Eldeshan W, Rutkowski E. COVID-19-related stroke. Translational Stroke Research. 2020;**11**(11):1-4. DOI: 10.1007/s12975-020-00818-9

[7] Paterson RW, Brown RL, Benjamin L, et al. The emerging spectrum of COVID-19 neurology: Clinical, radiological and laboratory findings. Brain (A Journal of Neurology). 2020. DOI: 10.1093/brain

[8] Brann DH, Tsukahara T, Weinreb C, et al. Non-neural expression of SARS-CoV-2 entry genes in the olfactory system suggests mechanisms underlying COVID-19-associated anosmia. Science Advances. 2020. DOI: 10.1126/sciadv.abc5801

[9] Nalbandian A, Sehgal K, Gupta A, et al. Post-acute COVID-19 syndrome. Nature Medicine. 2021;**27**:601-661. DOI: 10.1038/s41591-021-01283-z

[10] Godfred-Cato S, Bryant B, Leung J, et al. COVID-19-associated multisystem inflammatory syndrome in children—United States March-July 2020. Morbidity and Mortality Weekly Report. 2020;**69**(32):1074-1080. DOI: 10.15585/mmwr.mm6932e2

[11] World Health Organization. Coronavirus (Q&A)—Older People and COVID-19. Available from: www.who.int

[12] Santos de Oliveira MH, Lippi G, Henry BM. Sudden rise in COVID-19 case fatality among young and middle-aged adults in the south of Brazil after identification of the novel B.1.1.28.1 (P.1) SARS-CoV-2 strain: Analysis of data from the state of Parana. medRxiv. 2021. DOI: 10.1101/2021.03.24.21254046

[13] Richardson S, Hirsch JS, Narasimhan M, et al. Presenting characteristics, comorbidities, and outcomes among 5700 patients hospitalized with COVID-19 in the New York city area. Journal of the American Medical Association. 2020;**323**(20):2052-2059. DOI: 10.1001/jama.2020.6775

[14] Zheng Z, Peng F, Xu B, et al. Risk factors of critical & mortal COVID-19 cases: A systematic literature review and meta-analysis. Journal of Infection. 2020;**81**(2):e16-e25. DOI: 10.1016/j.jinf.2020.04.021

[15] Wichmann D, Sperhake J-P, Lutgehetmann M, et al. Autopsy findings and venous thromboembolism in patients with COVID-19; a prospective cohort study. Annals of Internal Medicine. 2020:M20-M2003. DOI: 10.7326/M20-2003

[16] Dai M, Liu D, Liu M, et al. Patients with cancer appear more vulnerable to SARS-CoV-2: A multicenter study during the COVID-19 outbreak. Cancer Discovery. 2020;**10**(6):783-701. DOI: 10.1158/2159-8290.CD-20-0422

[17] Ng J, Bakrania K, Falkous C, Russell R. COVID-19 Mortality Rates by Age and Gender: Why Is the Disease Killing More Men than Women? RGA; 2020

[18] Berlin I, Thomas D, Le Faou A-L, Cornuz J. COVID-19 and smoking. Nicotine and Tobacco Research. 2020;**22**(9):1650-1652. DOI: 10.1093/ntr/ntaa059

[19] Setti L, Passarini F, De Gennaro G, Barbieri P, Perone MG, Piazzalunga A, et al. The potential role of particulate matter in the spreading of COVID-19 in Northern Italy: First evidence-based research hypotheses. mediRxiv. 2020. DOI: 10.1101/2020.04.11.20061713

[20] Clerkin KJ, Fried JA, Raikhelkar J, Sayer G, Griffin JM, Masoumi A, et al. COVID-19 and cardiovascular disease. Circulation. 2020;**141**:1648-1655. DOI: 10.1161/CIRCULATIONAHA.120.046941

[21] Nguyen LH, Drew DA, Graham MS, et al. Risk of COVID-19 among front-line health-care workers and the general community: A prospective cohort study. The Lancet. 2020;**9**(5):e475-e483

[22] Bandyopadhyay S, Baticulon RE, Kadhum M, et al. Infection and mortality of healthcare workers worldwide from COVID-19: A systematic review. British Medical Journal Global Health. 2020;**5**:e003097

[23] Callaway E. Beyond Omicron: What's next for COVID's viral evolution. Nature. 2021;**600**:204-207. DOI: 10.1038/d41586-021-03619-8

[24] Mallapaty S. India's massive COVID surge puzzles scientists. Nature. 2021;**592**:667-668. DOI: 10.1038/d41586-021-01059-y

[25] Li B, Deng A, Li K, et al. Viral infection and transmission in a large, well-traced outbreak caused by the SARS-CoV-2 Delta variant. medRxiv. 2021. DOI: 10.1101/2021.07.07.21260122

[26] Urashima M, Otani K, Hasegawa Y, Akutsu T. BCG vaccination and mortality of COVID-19 across 173 countries: An ecological study. International Journal of Environmental Research and Public Health. 2020;**17**(15):5589. DOI: 10.3390/ijerph17155589

[27] Oh S, Shin JH, Jang EJ, et al. Anti-inflammatory activity of chloroquine and amodiaquine through p21-mediated suppression of T cell proliferation and Th1 cell differentiation. Biochemical and Biophysical Research Communications. 2016;**474**(2):345-350. DOI: 10.1016/j.bbrc.2016.04.105

[28] Águas R, Mahdi A, Shretta R, et al. Potential health and economic impacts of dexamethasone treatment for patients with COVID-19. Nature Communications. 2012;**12**:915. DOI: 10.1038/s41467-021-21134-2

[29] Pike JW, Christakos S. Biology and mechanisms of action of the vitamin D hormone. Endocrinology and Metabolism Clinics of North America. 2017;**46**(4):815-843. DOI: 10.1016/j.ecl.2017.07.001

[30] Ilie PC, Stefanescu S, Smith L. The role of vitamin D in the prevention of coronavirus disease 2019 infection and mortality. Aging Clinical and Experimental Research. 2020;**32**(7):1195-1198. DOI: 10.1007/s40520-020-01570-8

[31] Velthuis AJW, van den Worm SHE, Sims AC, Baric RS, Snider EJ, van Hemert MJ. Zn^{2+} inhibits coronavirus and arterivirus RNA polymerase activity in vitro and zinc ionophores block the replication of these viruses in cell culture. PLOS Pathogens. 2010. DOI: 10.1371/journal.ppat.1001176

[32] Gao Y, Yan L, Huang Y, Liu F-J, et al. Structure of the RNA-dependent RNA polymerase from COVID-19 virus. Science. 2020;**368**(6492):779-782. DOI: 10.1126/science.abb7498

[33] Pal A, Squitti R, Picozza M, et al. Zinc and COVID-19: Basis of current clinical trials [published online ahead of print, 2020 Oct 22]. Biological Trace Elements Research. 2020:1-11. DOI: 10.1007/s12011-020-02437-9

[34] Ruttkay-Nedecky B, Nejdl L, Gumulrc J, Zitka O, Masarik M, Eckschlager T, et al. The role of metallothionein in oxidative stress. International Journal of Molecular Sciences. 2013;**14**(3):6044-6066

[35] Siddoo-Atwal C. Chapter 17—Biological effects of uranium and its decay products on soil microbes, plants, and humans. In: Varma A, Tripathi S, Prasad R, editors. Plant Microbe Interface. Switzerland AG: Springer Nature; 2019. pp. 369-391

[36] Mayor-Ibarguren A, Busca-Arenzana C, Robles-Marhuenda Á. A hypothesis for the possible role of zinc in the immunological pathways related to COVID-19 infection. Frontiers in Immunology. 2020;**11**:1736. DOI: 10.3389/fimmu.2020.01736

[37] Finzi E. Treatment of SARS-CoV-2 with high dose oral zinc salts: A report on four patients. International Journal of Infectious Diseases. 2020;**98**:307-308. DOI: 10.1016/j.ijid.2020.06.006

[38] Prasad AS, Fitzgerald JT, Bao B, et al. Duration of symptoms and plasma cytokine levels in patients with the common cold treated with zinc acetate. A randomized, double-blind, placebo-controlled trial. Annals of Internal Medicine. 2000;**133**:245-252

[39] Kim Y, Kim H, Bae S, et al. Vitamin C is an essential factor on the anti-viral immune responses through the production of interferon-α/β at the initial stage of influenza A virus (H_3N_2) infection. Immune Network. 2013;**13**(2):70-74. DOI: 10.4110/in.2013.13.2.70

[40] Grosso G, Bei R, Mistretta A, Marventano S, Calabrese G, Masuelli L, et al. Effects of vitamin C on health: A review of evidence. Frontiers in Bioscience (Landmark Ed). 2013;**18**:1017-1029. DOI: 10.2741/4160

[41] Holford P, Carr AC, Jovic TH, et al. Vitamin C—an adjunctive therapy for respiratory infection, sepsis and COVID-19. Nutrients. 2020;**12**(12):3760. DOI: 10.3390/nu12123760

[42] Siddoo-Atwal C. A preliminary study of COVID-19 prevention through vitamin C, D, and zinc supplementation in a small clinic setting: Part I & II. Journal of Infectious Diseases and Research. 2021;**4**(S1):04

[43] Callaway E. Fast-spreading COVID variant can elude immune responses. Nature. 2022;**589**:500-501. DOI: 10.1038/d41586-021-00121-z

[44] Planas D, Saunders N, Maes P, et al. Considerable escape of

SARS-CoV-2 variant Omicron to antibody neutralization. bioRxiv. 2021. DOI: 10.1101/2021.12.14.472630

[45] Lu L, Bobo Mok BW-Y, Chen L-L, et al. Neutralization of SARS-CoV-2 Omicron variant by sera from BNT162b2 or Coronavac vaccine recipients. Clinical Infectious Diseases. 2021:ciab1041. DOI: 10.1093/cid/ciab1041

[46] Medigeshi G, Batra G, Murugesan DR, et al. Sub-optimal neutralisation of omicron (B.1.1.529) variant by antibodies induced by vaccine alone or SARS-CoV-2 infection plus vaccine (hybrid immunity) post 6-months. medRxiv. 2022. DOI: 10.1101/2022.01.04.22268747

[47] Ai J, Zhang H, Zhang Y, et al. Omicron variant showed lower neutralizing sensitivity than other SARS-CoV-2 variants to immune sera elicited by vaccines after boost. Emerging Microbes & Infections. 2021. DOI: 10.1080/22221751.2021.2022440

[48] Keeton R, Tincho MB, Ngomti A, et al. SARS-CoV-2 spike T cell responses induced upon vaccination or infection remain robust against Omicron. medRxiv. 2021. DOI: 10.1101/2021.12.26.21268380

[49] Gao Y, Cai C, Grifoni A, et al. Ancestral SARS-CoV-2-specific T cells cross-recognize the Omicron variant. Nature Medicine. 2022. DOI: 10.1038/s41591-022-01700-x

[50] Available from: https://www.fda.gov/vaccines-blood-biologics/safety-availability-biologics/thimerosal-

[51] Siddoo-Atwal C. Heavy metal carcinogenesis: A possible mechanistic role for apoptosis. Vegetos. 2017;**30**(Special):125-132. DOI: 10.5958/2229-4473.2017.00046.5

[52] Greinacher A, Thiele T, Warkentin TE, et al. A prothrombotic thrombocytopenic disorder resembling heparin-induced thrombocytopenia following coronavirus-19 vaccination. 2021. PREPRINT (Version 1) available at Research Square. DOI: 10.21203/rs.3.rs-362354/v1

[53] Remmel A. Why is it so hard to investigate the rare side effects of COVID vaccines? Nature. 2021. DOI: 10.1038/d41586-021-00880-9

[54] Taquet M, Dercon Q, Harrison PJ. Six-month sequelae of post-vaccination SARS-CoV-2 infection: A retrospective cohort study of 10,024 breakthrough infections. medRxiv. 2021. DOI: 10.1101/2021.10.26.21265508

[55] Katzourakis A. COVID-19: Endemic doesn't mean harmless. Nature. 2022;**601**:485. DOI: 10.1038/d41586-022-00155-x

Section 4

Infections with RNA Viruses

Chapter 5

Chronic Inflammatory Bowel Disease and Demyelination of the Central Nervous System: A Report on Two Cases

Oumerzouk Jawad, Klevor Raymond, Chraa Mohamed, Louhab Nissrine and Kissani Najib

Abstract

The objective of this article is to investigate the link between chronic inflammatory bowel disease (IBD) and central nervous system (CNS) demyelination. CNS demyelinating disorders in IBD are rare complications and are due to a dysimmune mechanism. We report the clinical cases of two patients followed for IBD. The first patient had Crohn's disease for 12 years and developed acute disseminated encephalomyelitis (ADEM) 1 month after the first course of the anti-tumor necrosis factor alpha (anti-TNF-alpha), infliximab. The second patient, treated for ulcerative colitis with salazopyrin, developed multiple sclerosis (MS) 5 months after the start of her disease. MS and optic neuritis remain the inflammatory demyelinating diseases of the CNS most frequently associated with IBD. The activation of T lymphocytes during IBD plays an essential role in the pathogenesis of MS and ADEM in a genetically predisposed population. It is currently recommended that patients with IBD be evaluated clinically and by MRI for subclinical demyelinating lesions in order to guide therapeutic management.

Keywords: chronic inflammatory bowel diseases, multiple sclerosis, encephalomyelitis

1. Introduction

1.1 Clinical case 1

We report the clinical history of a 45-year-old patient, followed up for 12 years for Crohn's disease. The patient was initially treated with sulfasalazine during the first 2 years of the disease and then, following an exacerbation of the disease, with azathioprine 100 mg/day and prednisolone 80 mg/day. The evolution was marked by a stabilization of the disease with the occurrence of complications of long-term corticosteroid therapy including adrenal insufficiency and steroid-induced diabetes for which he was placed on hydrocortisone and insulin therapy. However, given the persistence of active and fistulizing bowel involvement on thoraco-abdomino-pelvic computed tomography, the patient was started on anti-TNF-alpha (infliximab), after gradual reduction of oral corticosteroid therapy. The evolution was marked 1 month after the first infliximab treatment, by the rapidly progressive onset over 5 days, of weakness on the right side of his body with dysarthria, in a context of apyrexia without constitutional symptoms. The patient did not report any history of infection or vaccination in the month preceding the onset of this clinical picture. The neurological examination showed a spastic right hemiparesis, predominantly in the right lower limb with bilateral Babinski, and the fundus showed signs of periphlebitis in the peripheral retina. Brain MRI showed a left capsulo-thalamo-lenticular lesion with poorly defined margins, which appeared hypointense on T1 and hyperintense on T2, Fluid-attenuated inversion recovery (FLAIR), and diffusion sequences. The lesion was not enhanced after injection of contrast medium and exhibited hemorrhagic changes with significant perilesional edema exerting a discrete mass effect on the ventricular system. A second lesion was noted at the right capsulo-lenticular level, of smaller volume, also with hemorrhagic changes (**Figure 1**). The spectro-MRI data were compatible with an inflammatory process, and the angiographic sequences did not show venous thrombosis or signs of cerebral vasculitis. At this stage, in consultation with the neuroradiologist, we considered the diagnoses of acute disseminated encephalomyelitis (ADEM) and certain opportunistic infections, notably cerebral toxoplasmosis. The spinal cord MRI was unremarkable, and the lumbar puncture showed aseptic lymphocytic meningitis with 73 white blood cells/mm3 (100% lymphocytes), zero red blood cells, elevated Cerebrospinal fluid (CSF) proteins of 0.70 g/l, CSF glucose of 0.87 g/l (glycemia = 1.47 g/l) without intrathecal synthesis of immunoglobulins. Inflammatory and immunological tests, biopsy of the accessory salivary glands, angiotensin-converting enzyme assay, viral and toxoplasmosis serologies, PCR for *Mycobacterium tuberculosis,* and the rest of the biological workup were unremarkable. The diagnosis of ADEM associated with Crohn's disease was retained, and the patient received a bolus of methylprednisolone 500 mg/day for 6 days, followed by oral corticosteroid therapy (prednisolone 40 mg/day) with progressive tapering over 5 weeks. The clinical evolution was marked by the progressive recovery of muscle strength on the right side of the body, and the control brain MRI, 1 month after the halt of oral corticotherapy showed an almost complete disappearance of the lesions previously found. The biotherapy was stopped, and the decision to restart it was deferred.

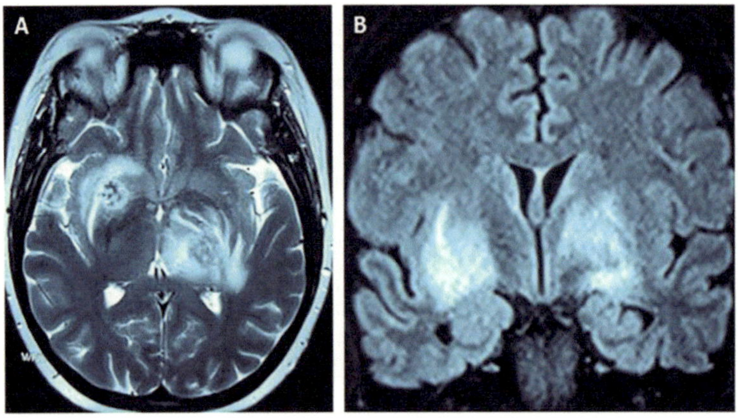

Figure 1.
Brain MRI, T2 (A) and FLAIR (B) sequences, showing bilateral and asymmetric, poorly demarcated T2 and Flair hyperintensities in the left thalamo-capsulo-lenticular and right capsulo-lenticular areas, with hemorrhagic changes.

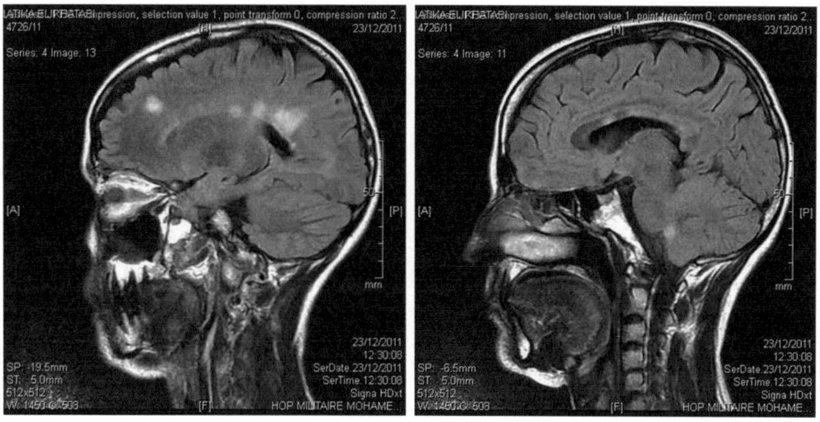

Figure 2.
Sagittal brain MRI, FLAIR sequence, showing multiple signal intensities involving the corpus callosum and inferior cerebellar peduncle.

1.2 Clinical case 2

This is a 32-year-old patient, followed for 5 months for ulcerative colitis under salazopyrin, and admitted to the emergency room with a gait instability of rapidly progressive onset over a week and accompanied by a rotatory vertigo. The patient also presented a spontaneously regressive episode of numbness with paresthesias of the left lower limb lasting 1 month. Clinical examination found a statokinetic cerebellar syndrome, a left lateralized central vestibular syndrome with a tetrapyramidal syndrome. The fundus was normal, and magnetic resonance imaging showed multiple T2 and FLAIR signal intensities of the white matter in the frontal, bilateral parietal, occipital, corpus callosum, and inferior cerebellar peduncle, without contrast (**Figure 2**). These radiological images were suggestive of a demyelinating disease such as multiple sclerosis (MS). The spinal cord MRI was unremarkable, and the lumbar puncture showed a clear fluid with two white blood cells/mm^3, zero red blood cells, a protein level of 0.24 g/l with intrathecal immunoglobulin synthesis; the visual evoked potentials were unremarkable. The immunological and inflammatory workup, as well as the rest of the biological workup, was unremarkable. The patient received a bolus of methylprednisolone at a dose of 3 g, then was placed on a disease-modifying treatment, interferon β 1a. The evolution was marked by the regression of the cerebellar syndrome and vertigo, without neurological or digestive relapse with an aborted progression of disease for 18 months.

2. Discussion

Neurological complications of idiopathic chronic inflammatory bowel disease (IBD), with an estimated prevalence between 47 and 50% depending on the series, normally appear after the diagnosis of IBD, coinciding or worsening with the exacerbation of IBD [1–3]. This neurological involvement is often related either to a dysimmune mechanism or to a prothrombotic state [4, 5]. However, multiple sclerosis (MS) and optic neuritis remain the most common inflammatory demyelinating diseases of the central nervous system (CNS) associated with IBD [1, 6, 7].

This is explained by the disruption of T cell function, as well as that of antigen-presenting cells, which is common between the two diseases [1, 2, 8, 9]. Therefore, cellular immune suppressive therapies are effective in treating both diseases [10, 11]. Activation of these T cells against the major determinants of myelin (myelin basic protein; MBP, proteolipid protein; PLP and myelin oligodendrocyte protein; MOG), through a mechanism of molecular mimicry (cross-immune response), also plays an essential role in the pathogenesis of ADEM [3, 4, 12].

In addition, proinflammatory cytokines (TNF-α, interleukin-2, and interferon-γ) associated with IBD may be a potential etiological factor in ADEM [4]. Therefore, IBD may represent a chronic pre-demyelinating condition and the equivalent of a triggering factor, and ADEM may represent an extraintestinal manifestation of IBD, through cross-autoimmunity [5, 11].

However, it is still initially difficult to differentiate between CNS involvement secondary to cerebral vasculitis lesions involving small vessels, cerebral venous thrombosis, and primary CNS demyelination associated with IBD [2, 3, 8, 9]. Cases of necrotizing vasculitis may result in forms similar to acute hemorrhagic encephalomyelitis, a variant of ADEM [5]. In addition, animal studies have shown that demyelinating lesions such as MS or ADEM in IBD patients correspond to lesions of cerebral venous thrombosis [3, 5, 9]. Perivenous demyelination is thought to be secondary to edema following blockage of venous drainage [11].

Finally, demyelinating lesions of the CNS pose a problem of differential diagnosis with demyelinating lesions secondary to the use of immunosuppressants and immunomodulators and with demyelinating lesions secondary to opportunistic infections in these immunocompromised patients [1–3, 8]. In fact, biotherapy (anti-TNF-alpha) may be responsible for the onset or worsening of CNS demyelinating disease in genetically predisposed individuals, opportunistic infections, or reactivation of latent infections, as well as thromboembolic complications and cerebral vasculitis [4, 7, 12]. The time interval between the start of anti-TNF-alpha administration and the onset of neurological symptoms is highly variable, with an average of 5 months [11]. In fact, TNF-alpha, which is a pro-inflammatory cytokine that plays a pivotal role in chronic inflammatory reactions in the gut and brain, is essential for CNS remyelination in the late stages of the disease through an anti-inflammatory action, and suppression of TNF-alpha action may therefore potentiate inflammation and demyelination [5, 8, 11]. It is currently advocated that before initiating anti-TNF-alpha therapy in patients with IBD, they should be well evaluated neurologically, clinically, and with MRI, for subclinical demyelinating lesions [12].

In conclusion, in our patient followed up for active Crohn's disease, ADEM could be secondary either to a cross-immune reaction coinciding with the worsening of IBD or a side effect of biotherapy, given the time interval between the beginning of treatment and the neurological symptoms. It would be plausible to stop the biotherapy and discuss other therapeutic alternatives.

Conflict of interest

The authors declare that they have no conflict of interest.

Author details

Oumerzouk Jawad[1,2,3]*, Klevor Raymond[2,3], Chraa Mohamed[2,3], Louhab Nissrine[2,3] and Kissani Najib[2,3]

1 Neurology Department, Mohamed V Military Training Hospital, Rabat, Morocco

2 Faculty of Medicine and Pharmacy of Marrakesh, Neuroscience Research Laboratory, Marrakesh, Morocco

3 Department of Neurology, Mohammed VI University Medical Center, Marrakesh, Morocco

*Address all correspondence to: tamamro@yahoo.fr

References

[1] Aziz M, Stivaros S, Fagbemi A, Vassallo G. Acute disseminated encephalomyelitis in conjunction with inflammatory bowel disease. European Journal of Paediatric Neurology. 2013;**17**(2):208-211

[2] Buzaglo G, Salleron J, Gower-Rousseau C, Wauquier N, Gonzales F, Vernier Massouille G, et al. MS/ICM association: Frequency and phenotype. Gastroentérologie Clinique et Biologique. 2009;**33**:296

[3] Kim J-M, Son C-N, Chang HW, Kim S-H. Simultaneous presentation of acute disseminated encephalomyelitis (ADEM) and systemic lupus erythematosus (SLE) after enteroviral infection: Can ADEM present as the first manifestation of SLE? Lupus. 2015;**24**(6):633-637

[4] Ordonez L, Skromne E, Ontaneda D, Rivera VM. Multiphasic disseminated encephalomyelitis, systemic lupus erythematosus and antiphospholipid syndrome. Clinical Neurology and Neurosurgery. 2007;**109**:102-105

[5] Scheid R, Teich N. Neurologic manifestations of ulcerative colitis. European Journal of Neurology. 2007; **14**(5):483-493

[6] Baumer FM, Ouahed J, Verhave M, Rivkin MJ. Fatal central nervous system disease following first infliximab infusion in a child with inflammatory bowel disease. Pediatric Neurology. 2016;**57**:91-94

[7] Scheid R, Teich N. Neurologic manifestations of ulcerative colitis. European Journal of Neurology. 2007; **14**:483-493

[8] Gupta G, Gelfand JM, Lewis JD. Inflammatory bowel disease: An increased risk factor for neurologic complications. Gastroenterology. 2005; **129**(3):819-826

[9] Casella G, Tontini GE, Bassotti G, Pastorelli L, Villanacci V, Spina L, et al. Neurological disorders and inflammatory bowel diseases. World Journal of Gastroenterology. 2014;**20**(27):8764-8782

[10] Stovicek J, Liskova P, Lisy J, Hlava S, Keil R. Crohn's disease: Is there a place for neurological screening? Scandinavian Journal of Gastroenterology. 2014; **49**(2):173-176

[11] Theibich A, Dreyer L, Magyari M, Locht H. Demyelinizing neurological disease after treatment with tumor necrosis factor alpha-inhibiting agents in a rheumatological outpatient clinic: Description of six cases. Clinical Rheumatology. 2014;**33**(5):719-723

[12] Gekka M, Sugiyama T, Nomura M, Kato Y, Nishihara H, Asaoka K. Histologically confirmed case of cerebral vasculitis associated with Crohn's disease—A case report. BMC Neurology. 2015;**15**:169

Chapter 6

Neurotropic Virus-Induced Meningoencephalomyelitis

Fareeha Saadi, Debanjana Chakravarty, Grishma Kasle and Jayasri Das Sarma

Abstract

Meningoencephalomyelitis emanates under the umbrella relating inflammatory changes of the Central Nervous System (CNS). Meningitis denotes inflammation in the meningeal layers, encephalitis is an acute diffuse inflammation of the brain, and inflammation in the spinal cord is denoted as myelitis. These can be interrelated or independent of each other depending on the etiology. The entire mechanism of meningoencephalomyelitis is governed by an acute innate inflammatory branch followed by a chronic progressive, adaptive branch of immunity with clinical signs like hyperthermia, weight loss, hypoxia, leukocytosis. This book chapter will focus on viral-induced meningitis, encephalitis, and myelitis. Thirty years of experience working with a murine-β-coronavirus (m-CoV); Mouse hepatitis virus (MHV)-A59 induced experimental model system provided us a thorough understanding of neuroglial cell-mediated acute neuroinflammation, denoted by the accumulation of leukocyte-common-antigen (LCA) positive or $CD45^+$ leukocytes in perivascular infiltrates referred to as perivascular cuff formation and microglial nodules in the brain parenchyma, which mimics specific pathology of human neurological disease multiple sclerosis (MS). Additionally, in this chapter, we summarized the role of CNS resident microglial activation and its interaction with peripheral migratory T cells in mounting neuropathogenesis and host immunity in different families of neurotrophic encephalomyelitis viruses that cause CNS inflammation.

Keywords: meningioencephalomyelitis, demyelination, axonal loss, murine-β-coronavirus (m-CoV), neuroinflammation, multiple sclerosis (MS)

1. Introduction

Encephalitis is a pathological entity that refers to the inflammation of the *encephalon* or the brain parenchyma due to infection, autoimmunity, and brain injury. It is a rare medical condition with clinically serious consequences ranging from headaches, fever, seizures, permanent disability, and brain damage. Encephalitis majorly affects infants and the elderly above the age of 65, whereas, the incidence is transitional in the youth and is of significant public health importance because of the associated morbidity and mortality [1]. It results in varied clinical symptoms, such as mild fever and headaches to severe cognitive impairment accompanied by loss of physical vigor and unconsciousness or even life-threatening symptoms that can result in permanent brain damage [2, 3]. It is believed that the severe inflammation associated with encephalitis causes swelling in the brain, which in turn gives rise to headaches, stiff neck, mental confusion, and even seizures [1, 4]. Though cases are recognized in all populations and ages, pediatric populations, young adults, and especially males have a higher propensity to encephalitis [5–7].

Infection by a virus is the most common and important cause of encephalitis [8]. Virus infections can also cause aseptic meningitis and myelitis [9, 10]. Research on viral encephalitis has gained much momentum with the recognition of encephalitis in human immunodeficiency virus (HIV) infection of the CNS and the emerging viruses such as West Nile virus (WNV), Nipah virus, and severe acute respiratory syndrome viruses (SARS-CoV and SARS-CoV-2) [11]. Members of several virus families like flaviviruses, paramyxoviruses, alphaviruses, bunyaviruses, orthomyxoviruses, arenaviruses, enteroviruses, rhabdoviruses, and astroviruses are also known to cause encephalitis [12].

Viruses may directly enter into the CNS or replicate away from the CNS at first and gain entry to the CNS through various routes [13, 14]. Local factors, like pH, mucosal immune responses, or the integrity of skin and mucosal barriers, govern the entry of the virus into the CNS and resultant encephalitis. Virus entry and replication activate the CNS resident immune cells, which, together with peripheral leukocytes, induce host immune response and promote encephalitis and neuroinflammation, resulting in multiple changes to the CNS physiology [15]. Histopathologically, characteristic microglial nodule formation, i.e., the accumulation of activated microglia in the brain parenchyma and the perivascular cuff formation, is observed in encephalitic brains [16–18]. Once the virus clears, the acute behavioral symptoms are resolved; however, long-term psychiatric, neurocognitive, and degenerative issues persist due to the ongoing immune responses in the CNS even after pathogen clearance [18, 19].

Interestingly, people infected with neurotropic viruses may not always develop encephalitis, indicating that host cell factors may play a critical role in regulating the outcome of the disease process. While mounting shreds of evidence are available to understand these host factors, limited information is available to understand the genomic control of the pathogenic properties and host factors that mediate a balance between neurovirulence and neuroprotection. Host cell response pathways like UPR and ER stress and oxidative stress may alter due to robust viral replication and intracellular assembly, causing imbalance between reactive oxygen species and antioxidants. These are governed by a battery of cellular mediators like DJ-1, Nrf-2, catalase, HMOX, MMPs, NADPH oxidase, cytokines, chemokines, and secondary messengers. These mediators are either CNS resident proteins or may be produced by the CNS resident neuro-glial cells like microglia, astrocytes, endothelial cells, and peripherally derived leukocytes that enter the CNS upon inflammation and breaching of the blood-brain barrier [13]. The nexus of these immune-inflammatory mediators with endogenous host proteins are well studied for ages in mounting host immunity. The question lies in whether host immunity plays a protective or pathogenic role.

Moreover, understanding the inflammatory mechanisms of meningioencephalomyelitis is a challenge in human patients due to the unavailability of the high throughput data from non-invasive techniques like MRI, fMRI, CT, and detailed invasive histopathological data from punched-biopsy/autopsy tissues. Thus, a thorough understanding of the cellular factors ranging from genomic control of pathogenic properties to viral host factors and immunomodulatory effects requires cause-effect relationship experimental animal models/systems that can provide detailed insight into the disease process instrumental in the diagnosis and designing therapeutics. Though the use of mouse models to understand human disease has its limitations, critical pathological features of encephalitis can be efficiently reproduced in viral-induced experimental models. This book chapter will majorly summarize studies on viral encephalitis and its consecutive neuroinflammatory demyelination and axonal loss.

2. Routes of infection emanating to neurotropic virus infection

The term "neurotropic" refers to affinity towards the nervous system and displays the properties of neuroinvasion (entry into the CNS), and has direct neuroglial tropism. The viral entry to the neuroglial cells may be via receptor-mediated endocytosis and its fusion with the cell cytoplasm. It may also enter via direct endocytosis irrespective of engaging a receptor. Mounting shreds of evidence reported that neurotropic virus enters the brain parenchyma from the olfactory epithelium or retinal ganglionic cells via retrograded axonal transport. Upon entry to the brain parenchyma, infectious virus particles may also follow anterograde axonal transport via the optic nerve to reach retinal ganglionic cells and also can spread to different anatomic regions of the brain like the hippocampus, cortex, anterior commissure, basal forebrain, amygdala, brain stem as well as down the spinal cord. The neurotropic viruses can also travel through the lung-brain axis and cause inflammation in the brain stem region, the respiratory center. Neurotropic viruses can also access brain parenchyma via the gut-brain axis through the vagus nerve.

3. Neurotropic virus infection in mice is employed as an experimental model system to understand the underlying mechanisms of encephalitis, poliomyelitis, neuroinflammation, and demyelination concurrent with axonal loss

Neuroinflammation is responsible for initiating direct neuroglial dystrophy, which in turn can activate CNS resident microglia to release immune modulators. Microglia, the major resident immune cells in the central nervous system (CNS), are considered as the key cellular mediators of neuroinflammatory processes. Microglial research has become a central focus in cellular neuroimmunology and neuroinflammation in the past few years. Chronic/remitting neurological disease such as multiple sclerosis (MS) has long been considered an inflammatory autoimmune disease with the infiltration of peripheral myelin-specific T cells into the CNS. With the rapid advancement in the field of microglia and astrocytic neurobiology, the term neuroinflammation progressively started to denote chronic CNS cell-specific inflammation in MS. The direct glial responses in MS are different from conventional peripheral immune responses. This book chapter attempts to summarize current findings of neuroinflammatory responses within the CNS by direct infection of neural cells by mouse hepatitis virus (MHV) and the mechanisms by which glial cell responses ultimately contribute to the meningioencephalomyelitis and demyelination concurrent with axonal loss (**Figure 1**). Microglia can be persistently infected by MHV. Microglial activation and phagocytosis are recognized to be critically important in the pathogenesis of

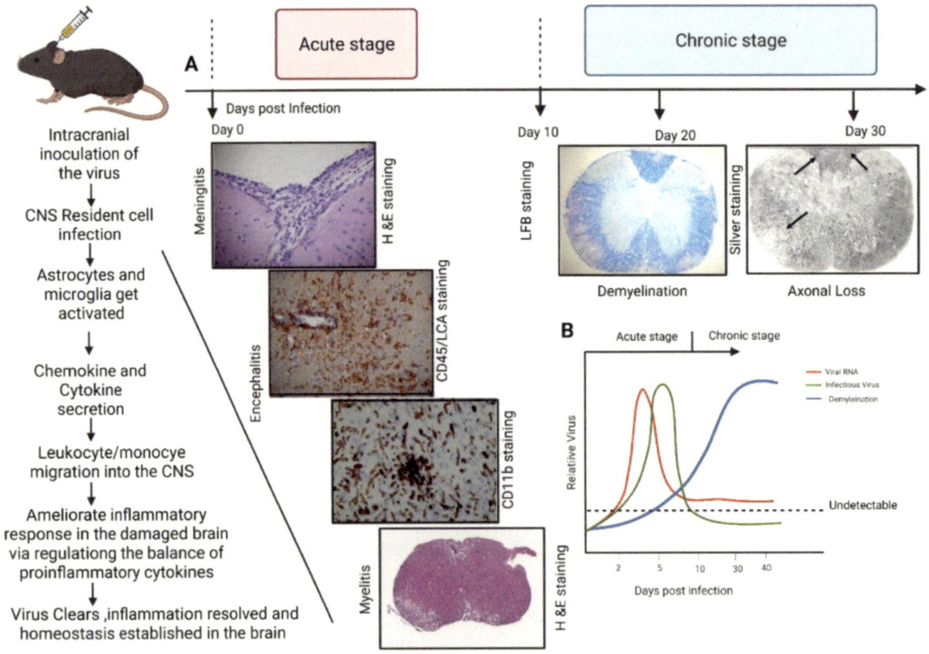

Figure 1.
Disease kinetics and pathological manifestations of murine β-CoV, MHV-A59 intracranial inoculation in C57BL/6 mice, a model to understand viral induced meningioencephalomyelitis and demyelination concurrent with axonal loss. (A) Shows the timeline of infection namely acute stage and its corresponding neuropathologies: meningitis denoting inflammation in the meningeal layers, encephalitis,an acute diffuse inflammation of the brain, and inflammation in the spinal cord denoted as myelitis and chronic progressive demyelination characterized by myelin loss concurrent with axonal loss. (B) Kinetics of MHV-A59 replication and viral clearance represented by viral RNA and infectious viral particles respectively and occurrence of demyelination [20].

demyelination. Emerging evidence for the pathogenic role of microglia and the activation of inflammatory pathways in these cells in MHV infection supports the concept that microglia-induced neuroinflammation is an amplifier of virus-induced neuropathology. Conventional understanding was that the peripheral immune cells are the major players for mounting CNS inflammatory responses. But the current studies revealed that if microglial activation and its immune modulators can check the infection, then the peripheral immune system need not be involved in mounting host immunity, and meningioencephalomyelitis may not shadow. In most cases, CNS resident microglial activation sets the stage for innate immune inflammation that results in the proinflammatory milieu of cytokines and chemokines, known as cytokine storm, which, while trying to combat pathogens, also causes damage to the CNS tissues. Amelioration of the proinflammatory condition requires anti-inflammatory cytokines where the peripheral immune system plays a major role. A series of recent studies on neurotropic murine β-coronavirus demonstrated acute-innate neuroinflammation mediated by CNS resident microglial interplay with peripheral leucocytes comprising monocytes and neutrophils NKT cells, $CD4^+$ and $CD8^+$ T cells to eradicate the pathogen and protect host tissue against aberrant tissue damage (**Figure 2**). In the below-mentioned sections of this book chapter, we are discussing in detail MHV infection as a prototype of β-coronavirus infection and its pathogenesis to understand the underpinning mechanism of meningioencephalomyelitis, demyelination and axonal loss.

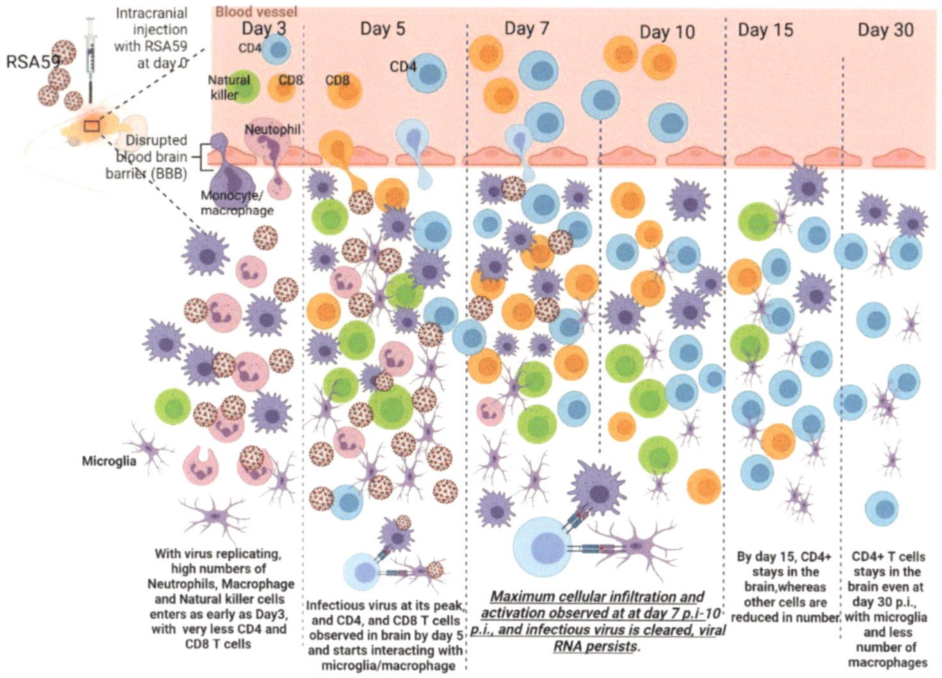

Figure 2.
Temporal kinetics of CNS resident glial cell activation associated with peripheral cell migration in response to RSA59 infection in the mouse CNS is key to cause meningioencephalomyeltits. Intracranial inoculation of RSA59 directly infects CNS resident neuroglial cells that in-turn activates CNS resident immune-glial cells like astrocytes and microglia. Activated CNS resident cells secrete a large number of inflammatory mediators like pro-inflammatory cytokines and chemokines. Microglial activation and its pro-inflammatory mileu in the inflamed CNS make a chemoattractant gradient to help the migration of peripheral leukocytes in the CNS. A differential infiltration of total myeloid (neutrophils, macrophages/monocytes, and microglia) and lymphoid (CD4, CD8, and NKT) cell populations observed at different time post infection is critical for orchestration of the clearance of the viral particle mounting host immunity by balancing the pro-inflammatory condition with the anti-inflammatory condition and restoring the CNS homeostasis.

3.1 MHV

Mouse hepatitis virus (MHV) is a β-CoV of the family Coronaviridae. It poses no threat to humans but shows similarities with other human viruses of the same family, such as SARS-CoV, MERS-CoV, and SARS-CoV-2 though they are evolutionarily distinct. MHV can infect the CNS and cause white matter lesions, which makes it an excellent viral model of neuroinflammatory demyelinating disease. Depending on the inoculation route and the strain of MHV-CoV, different outcomes are expected [21].

For example, a highly neurovirulent strain of MHV, JHM, J2.2-V-1, upon intracranial inoculation, induces a monophasic disease course, characterized by inflammatory cell infiltrates in the CNS with subsequent demyelination and clinical symptoms of hind limb weakness, ataxia, and paralysis [22, 23]. No auto-reactive T cells have ever been found in the CNS of J2.2-V-1-infected mice, and the disease is the resultant of virus-specific T cells, which indicated that virus alone can cause myelin destruction. Earlier it was believed that demyelination in JHM infection may be solely due to the lytic oligodendrocyte infection [24], but with the application of immune-deficient animal models, it became clear that immune-mediated mechanisms may be more important [25].

MHV-A59, a hepatotropic and neurotropic MHV strain, caused demyelination in C57BL/6 mice even in the absence of B and T cells [20]. The disease upon MHV-A59 intracranial administration also follows a biphasic course, where encephalomyelitis is characteristic of an acute phase peaking during days 5/6 post infection (p.i.) and chronic stage where demyelination and axonal degeneration peak on day 30 p.i. [26–29]. Thus, it can be said that different, but related MHV strains may induce demyelination via distinct mechanisms. MHV-A59 induced neuroinflammation and neuroimmune modulation mediated neuroglial dystrophy is triggered by the activation of cellular censors like Toll-like receptor (TLRs)/Rig-I-like receptor (RLRs)/synthase for the second messenger cyclic GMP-AMP and the cyclic GMP-AMP receptor stimulator of interferon genes (cGAS-STING) which can further activate the interferon regulatory factors (IRFs), nuclear factor kappa-light-chain-enhancer of activated B cells (NF-κB) and downstream type I interferon (IFN) genes. Acute-innate neuroinflammation is rather dependent on the CNS resident immune cell activation in association with peripheral derived myeloid cells, which in turn involve lymphoid cells in ameliorating proinflammatory condition and bring the anti-inflammatory condition in order to restore the homeostasis of the CNS compartment [30].

Studies are focused on understanding mechanisms from cellular sensing to the disease outcome comprising the MHV-A59 induced neuroinflammation encompassing encephalitis and microglial nodule formation and its progressive myelin pathology concurrent with axonal pathology. We have used and compared spike gene recombinant strains of MHV, a demyelinating strain (DM) RSA59, and non-demyelinating strain (NDM) RSMHV2 to understand the genomic control of encephalitic properties. A plethora of studies from the eminent scientists in this field, along with ours, have contributed to understanding the pathogenesis of MHV infection. Strains of MHV can cause direct CNS cell infection or access the CNS via retrograde axonal transport, but irrespective of the route, they cause encephalitis [31–33].

3.1.1 Comparative studies between spike gene recombinants murine coronaviruses RSA59 and RSMHV2 to understand the genomic control of meningioencephalomyelitic properties

Using targeted RNA recombination, two isogenic spike protein recombinant strains of MHV, RSA59, and RSMHV2 (background is from demyelinating strain MHV-A59) were generated. For RSA59, the spike was taken from the parental demyelinating strain MHV-A59, and RSMHV2 had the spike from the parental non-demyelinating MHV-2 strain. Enhanced green fluorescent protein (EGFP) was also inserted in the recombinants by replacing the nonessential gene 4a and part of 4b in the MHV-A59 genome by heterologous targeted recombination [34].

Comparative studies between the two recombinants revealed similar pathology to their parental strains for RSA59 and RSMHV2, respectively. Intracerebral (IC) inoculation of RSA59 in 4-week-old C57BL/6 mice caused acute hepatitis, neuroinflammation comprising of meningitis, encephalitis, myelitis, and chronic demyelination and axonal loss, characterized by lymphocytic infiltrates and microglial nodules with focal neuronophagia associated lepto-meningitis [29, 35]. IC inoculation of RSMHV2 caused acute stage hepatitis, meningitis, and encephalitis but no myelitis or chronic demyelination. The encephalitis was indeed more robust compared to RSA59. MHV-2 does not induce encephalitis; it cannot even enter the brain parenchyma and restricts to the meninges inducing meningitis alone [34].

Both RSA59 and RSMHV2 showed similar infection in the brain where they successfully infected and replicated in meninges, the site of inoculation (near the lateral geniculate nucleus), ventral striatum/basal forebrain, hippocampus, and brainstem, and infect the neurons, astrocytes, microglia, and oligodendrocytes in the brain. However, they show different tropism in the spinal cord. DM infects the grey matter neurons and takes an axonal route to be released at the nerve end, whereas in the white matter, it preferentially infects oligodendrocytes [36]. By day 7 p.i. most of the viruses have traversed to the spinal cord white matter. Though NDM can also infect the neurons in the grey matter, they fail to infect the white matter oligodendrocytes [35, 36] due to their inefficiency to translocate through neurites and fusion at the nerve end [37]. The difference in the disease outcome can be attributed to their differential spinal cord tropism and persistence. Thus, it can be inferred that the combined action of spike mediated axon transport of DM strain to evade the heightened immune response and ability to infect the white matter oligodendrocytes and persist in the white matter could be the key to inducing demyelination and axonal loss during the chronic phase of neuroinflammation. DM strain-induced axonal loss and myelin loss are associated with profuse accumulation of macrophages filled with myelin debris within the demyelinating plaques which is not observed in NDM strain infection. High resolution TEM microscopy revealed that microglia/macrophages are indeed responsible for direct myelin stripping, leading to demyelination [29, 35, 38].

It is important to note that neuroinflammation and encephalitis in MHV infection is accompanied with pronounced activation of CNS resident immune cells, microglia, and astrocytes. Upon activation, they take their characteristic activated phenotype and start expressing microglia/macrophage-specific protein Iba1 (ionized calcium-binding adaptor molecule 1), which promotes ruffling and phagocytosis [20, 38]. Detailed Affymetrix microarray analysis revealed that both RSA59 and RSMHV2 initiate innate immune responses during the acute phase with the expression of chemokines like CXCL10, CXCL9, CCL5, and CCL12 and other CD molecules that represent activation of microglia/macrophages [39]. Results also showed the induction of antiviral host response represented by the expression of perforins and IFN gamma signaling genes. Together, the acute stage innate-immune responses and encephalitis were comparable in both RSA59 and RSMHV2 infection [39].

The inflammatory responses gradually declined in RSMHV2 infection following virus clearance, but RSA59 chronic infection showed persistent microglia in the demyelinating plaques and the production of microglia-associated inflammatory mediators. Studies have shown that IFN responses can promote phagolysosomes maturation and autophagy in the persistently activated microglia/macrophages, which can promote myelin sheath engulfment leading to demyelination. This evidence demonstrated that RSA59 induced demyelination could occur through innate immune neuroinflammation denoted by meningioencephalomyelitis triggered during the acute infection stage. Although innate immune responses contribute partially towards controlling of initial virus spread, virus-specific T cell effector functions are essential to eliminate the infectious virus load during most acute infections. Control of m-CoV spread requires the functioning of both $CD4^+$ and $CD8^+$ T cells [40]. $CD8^+$ T cells are the primary effectors but require support from $CD4^+$ T cells. A recent study in $CD4^{-/-}$ mice showed impaired RSA59 clearance, despite the presence of functional $CD8^+$ T cells, demonstrating the importance of $CD4^+$ T cells for the efficient functioning of $CD8^+$ T responses [41].

The distinct cause-effect relationship-driven studies demonstrate that RSA59 infection can be instrumental towards understanding a direct CNS resident immune cell-mediated as well as antibody-mediated encephalomyelitis and demyelination pathologies.

Both DM and NDM strains show a reduction in the expression of genes responsible for innate immune response, and this reduction is more pronounced in the NDM strain-infected mice. In contrast, the genes involved in adaptive immune cell response are upregulated only in DM strain, specifically during the chronic stage of spinal cord infection. A significant upregulation of genes involved in T helper cell signaling pathways, B-cell development, and communication between innate and adaptive immune cells as well as of the expression of IgG genes are observed in the DM strain infection leading to chronic pathology but not in NDM strain [42].

While MHV infection in mouse is a prototype to understand the cellular and molecular consequences of encephalitis and demyelination, Theiler's murine encephalomyelitis virus (TMEV) in SJL mice also serves as another excellent experimental model of MS because of its histopathological and immunological similarities with MS.

3.2 Theiler's murine encephalomyelitis virus (TMEV) induced encephalitis

TMEV is a non-enveloped, single-stranded positive-sense RNA virus belonging to the family Picornaviridae and also used as a model to understand the immune-mediated mechanism of demyelination [43, 44].

Upon intracranial (i.c.) infection in SJL mice induces characteristic polioencephalomyelitis in the CNS. In a biphasic CNS disease, first, during the acute phase immune cells including the $CD4^+$ T cells and $CD8^+$ T cells infiltrate the CNS in response to profuse virus replication, and inflammation [45]. They exert rather protective effects by helping clear the virus from the grey matter and result in immune-mediated encephalomyelitis [46]. During the chronic phase, TMEV persistently infects glial cells and macrophages in the white matter, further, there is an infiltration of leukocytes, including macrophages, TMEV-specific T cells and antibodies. The immune effectors ($CD4^+$ and $CD8^+$ T cells) that exerted protective functions during the acute phase exert detrimental effects in the chronic phase by participating in epitope spreading to myelin antigens resulting in severe immune pathology in the white matter of the spinal cords, which causes demyelination [47]. White matter lesions harbor monocytes/macrophages and a few B cells in addition to the T lymphocytes [48]. Initially, the $CD4^+$ T cells recognized the abundant myelin protein PLP, but later, the $CD4^+$ T cells subsets start to recognize subdominant myelin protein epitopes and led to autoreactivity [47]. Additionally, the $CD8^+$ T cells have also been suggested to function as autoreactive cytotoxic cells or regulatory cells in TMEV infection [49]. TMEV induced CNS pathology is immunologically mediated like in MS, wherein MHC plays an important role, and substantial similarities exist in neuropathology, including axonal damage and remyelination [43]. Also, like MS, T-cell apoptosis is less in TMEV induced disease [50].

Cytokines are known to play important functions in the induction and regulation of immune responses against the neurotropic virus. Similarly, the cytokine production by the CNS resident cells astrocytes and microglia, as well as the peripheral immune cells such as T cells and macrophages heavily, influence the encephalitic response induced by TMEV infection [51, 52]. Studies have shown that a critical balance between the inflammatory cytokines governing the propagation of antiviral response to clear the virus during early infection and controlling of immune pathology and establish homeostasis during the late stage. That being said, no particular cytokine pattern is yet established and successfully associated with resistance or susceptibility to TMEV-induced encephalitis and demyelination by the different strains of the virus. A study compared the cytokine response between TMEV DA-infected susceptible (SJL) and resistant (B6) mice. Results showed a high expression of proinflammatory cytokines (IFN-γ, TNF-α, IL-1, IL-2, and IL-6) and low levels of anti-inflammatory cytokines (IL-4, IL-5, and IL-10) in the brains of both SJL and B6 mice during the early acute phase decreasing thereafter [51]. However, only in the SJL mice after a peak of the inflammatory response during day 8–12 p.i. in the brain with a minimum recorded during days 20–25 p.i., the second wave of inflammatory cytokine production was observed later in the spinal cord, which could explain the inflammatory demyelination only in the SJL mice. TGF-β, an important anti-inflammatory cytokine, has shown a significantly higher upregulation in SJL mice compared to B6 [51]. TGF-β can specifically inhibit the cytotoxic T lymphocyte (CTL) response [53] which is noted to be significantly impaired in the SJL mice resulting in reduced TMEV clearance and persistence, leading to virus-mediated encephalitis and demyelination.

4. Overview of microglial activation in encephalomyelitis: amplifier of virus-induced neuropathology

In the context of viral encephalitis that is characterized by an inflammatory response with meningeal, perivascular, and parenchymal infiltrates of peripheral leukocytes, studies have revealed that microglial activation acts as a double-edged sword [16]. On the one hand they promote multiple antiviral functions; microglia sense the ATP released by virus-infected neurons through the purinergic receptor P2Y12 and quickly migrate towards the infected neurons to exert their phagocytic activity [54]. They directly exert their antiviral effect by producing type 1 interferon (IFN-1), inducing IFN-stimulated gene (ISG) to activate corresponding signaling pathways [55]. Additionally, microglia induce autophagy and secrete cytokines to clear the virus from the tissue [56–58]. On the other hand, their persistent activation leads to tissue damage due to autophagy and apoptotic pathway activation, presynaptic membrane damage in the hippocampus mediated by the complement system activation, which further results in long-term memory impairment and cognitive dysfunction in patients with viral encephalitis [59–62].

The most common and important example of virus-induced chronic brain infection is the HIV [63]. HIV-induced encephalitis is typified by the accumulation of activated microglia in nodules-like phenotype throughout the parenchyma [64, 65]. HIV enters the CNS via the myelomonocytic cells such as monocytes, perivascular cells, and microglia [66]. HIV particularly targets and disables microglia in the CNS and T cells in the periphery, the key players in neuroinflammation [64, 67]. In fact, the persistence of HIV in microglia indicates that the virus uses the cells as the reservoir [68]. Even though reports suggest that microglia may perform protective functions early on during HIV infections, their functions are considerably compromised. Most studies suggest that active infection of microglia results in their secretion of a variety of neurotoxins, increasing neural apoptosis and neuronal autophagy [16]. Astrogliosis is another characteristic pathology following microglial activation that, together with microgliosis, ultimately leads to myelin paleness and neuronal loss. Patients with advanced AIDS are likely to develop severe encephalitis upon human cytomegalovirus

(HCMV) infection [69, 70]. HCMV infection is characterized by microglial nodular encephalitis consisting of microglia, astrocytes, and giant cells, and ventriculoencephalitis and is the main cause of dementia in AIDS patients [71].

Microglia are susceptible to congenital Zika virus (ZIKV) infection [61]. Histopathological analysis showed that ZIKV infects and activates microglia in the perivascular regions causing localized neuroinflammation [61]. Further, the virus is disseminated throughout the parenchyma, which is later associated with neuron damage, especially in the cortical regions [72]. Pronounced neuronal injury results in microcephaly noted in many cases of congenital ZIKV infection [72].

E3 ubiquitin ligase pellino (pelia) expressed by microglia promotes the replication of West nile virus (WNV) in microglia and neurons [73]. It also induces NF-κB and/or p38-MAPK signaling in the microglia that causes an upregulation of inflammatory cytokines and chemokines, leading to peripheral leukocytes infiltration [73, 74]. The robust neuroinflammation may lead to lethal WNV encephalitis.

It is interesting to note that many viruses from diverse families of viruses have been studied in microglia depletion models. Results from most studies showed increased viral replication upon microglial depletion [16, 75–77]. Additionally, microglial depletion was also associated with overt neurological symptoms and/or death along with high viral burden, which indicated their importance in survival in encephalitis [77]. Though confirmatory results on how these protective functions are exerted by microglia are lacking, some studies show a dependence of T cell responses on microglia activation.

Studies on several mouse models of viral encephalitis have shown that viral clearance depends on efficient T cell responses, including WNV, MHV, and TMEV [78–81]. TMEV model shows strain-specific differences in disease phenotype and viral clearance, which was associated with underlying differences in $CD8^+$ T cell responses subject to Treg suppression [82, 83]. Further investigation revealed that microglia depletion did not impact $CD8^+$ T cell recruitment but resulted in increased infiltration of Tregs, which caused clinical severity in C57BL/6 mice which is normally not susceptible to TMEV induced disease [84]. In the MHV-induced neuroinflammation model, both $CD8^+$ and $CD4^+$ T cells are implicated in viral clearance, but $CD4^+$ T cells have also been reported to contribute to pathogenesis [80, 85, 86]. A study showed that microglial depletion in mice infected with JHMV strain of MHV, rJ2.2 significantly reduced the infiltration of $CD4^+$ T cells and Tregs in the CNS along with a significant reduction in IFN-γ expression by $CD4^+$ T cells, but there was no impact on the $CD8^+$ T cell population [77]. Thus, showing the importance of microglia in especially orchestrating virus-specific $CD4^+$ T cell response.

In addition to these studies using the JHMV strain, MHV-A59 or its isogenic recombinant strain RSA59 have also elucidated a critical communication between microglia and $CD4^+$ T cell response. Using a $CD4^{-/-}$ mice model very recent study demonstrated for the first time that the mice are highly susceptible to RSA59 induced chronic demyelination with axonal loss [80]. Though the overall inflammation was not affected during the early time-points (day 5–6) i.e., the acute neuroinflammation phase, the CD11b + microglial activation was significantly impaired. The entire inflammatory response was skewed towards an M2 type which was also reflected in the persistence of characteristic amoeboid shaped phagocytic microglia in the CNS of the mice during the chronic phase (day 30 p.i.). Encephalitis, which usually resolves after the acute phase in RSA59 infection, persisted for as long as day 30 p.i. The brain stems of $CD4^{-/-}$ mice were populated with CD11b + microglia surrounding bulbar vacuolated pathology, which signified axonal death and damage [80]. Additionally,

$CD4^+$ T cell deficiency resulted in severe grey matter inflammation in the form of poliomyelitis in the spinal cords as well as the dorsal root ganglion (**Figure 3**). Together these results showed a critical interdependence of microglia and $CD4^+$ T cells in RSA59 infection. Typically, M2 microglial activation fails to resolve during the chronic infection, rendering mice more susceptible to demyelination and axonal bulbar vacuolation [80].

A very recent study on neurotropic coronavirus MHV-RSA59 infection in $Ifit2^{-/-}$ mice revealed that Ifit2 protects mice from uncontrolled replication and spread throughout the brain parenchyma as well as the spinal cord. Ifit2 deficiency showed pronounced morbidity and mortality in RSA59 infected mice. Furthermore, microglial activation in the CNS was impaired in infected $Ifit2^{-/-}$ mice compared to WT infected mice, and as a consequence, peripheral lymphocyte specifically NK1.1 T

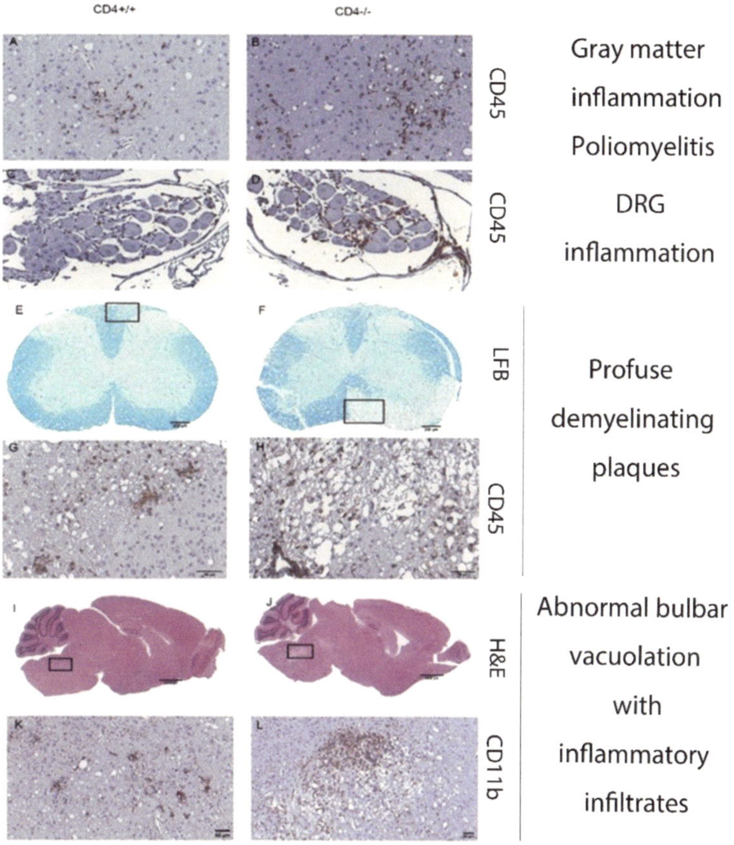

Figure 3.
CD4 deficiency causes poliomyelitis and the dorsal root ganglionic inflammation at acute phase and abnormal bulbar vacuolation at chronic phase of RSA59 infection. Serial sections of spinal cord, dorsal root ganglion and brain from $CD4^{+/+}$ and $CD4^{-/-}$ mouse were immunostained with anti-CD45, LFB and/or H&E. CD45 immunostining showed heightened poliomyelitis/inflammation of gray matter and inflammation of the dorsal root ganglia in the $CD4^{-/-}$ mice compared to $CD4^{+/+}$ mice at the acute phase of infection. Spinal cord sections form these mice when further analyzed at chronic stage for demyelination by LFB showed increased myelin loss in $CD4^{-/-}$ mice compared to $CD4^{+/+}$ mice, CD45 + inflammatory cells were observed in demyelinating lesions of both wildtype and CD4 deficient mice but were elevated in case of $CD4^{-/-}$ mice. Sagittal sections of the brain at chronic stage, stained with H&E showed large number of vacuoles in the brain stem region denoting abnormal bulbar vacuolation which was populated with and Cd11b + micgrogila/monocyte macrophages. Adapted from Chakravarty et al [41].

cells and CD4+ T cells migration to the CNS was restricted in the Ifit2$^{-/-}$ mice possibly contributing to the lack of viral clearance. Impaired microglial activation and reduced migration of inflammatory cells in the CNS may be associated with less encephalitis and devoid of mounting host immunity. These deficiencies were associated with a lower level of microglial expression of CX3CR1, the cognate receptor of the CX3CL1 (fractalkine) chemokine, which plays a critical role in both microglial activation and leukocyte recruitment. These findings highlighted a pivotal role of interferon stimulating genes and its tetratricopeptide protein as host cell factors in the induction of encephalitis and uncovered a new potential role of an interferon-induced protein in immune protection (**Figure 4**) [30].

Taking the above-mentioned experimental evidence of the role of CD4+ T cells and monocyte/macrophage activation in viral-induced neuroinflammation, further studies were geared to explore the interactome between the CD4+ T cell expressed CD40 Ligand and CD40 expressed on microglia. CD40-CD40L dyad is an important immune dyad that controls both CD4+ T cell and microglia functions [87, 88]. Our studies in CD40L$^{-/-}$ mice showed that the absence of CD40L renders mice highly susceptible to RSA59 infection due to reduced microglia/macrophage activation during the acute phase of infection required to eliminate the virus (**Figure 5**) [89]. Effector CD4+ T recruitment to the CNS is significantly dampened, and due to the

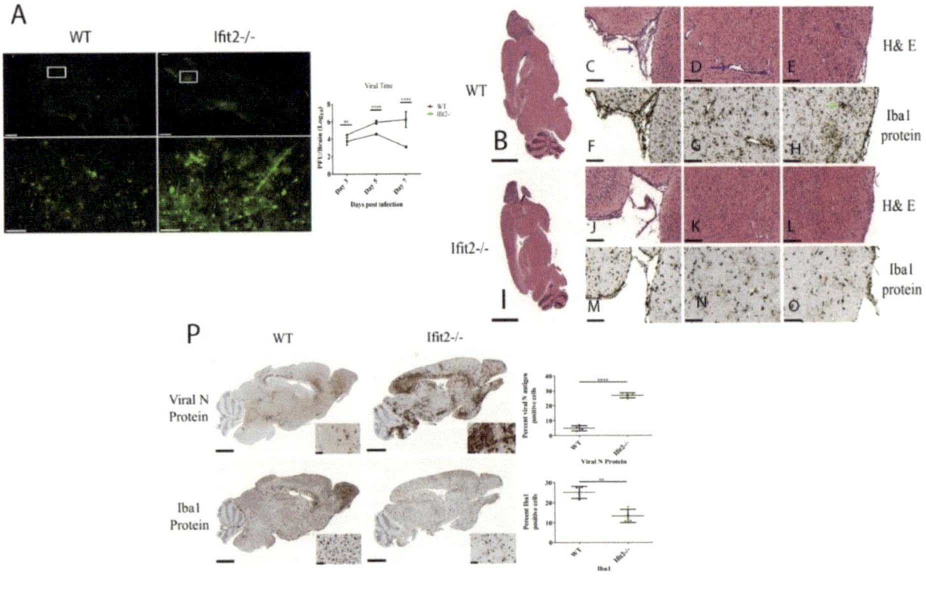

Figure 4.
Ifit2$^{-/-}$ mice upon a murine β-CoV RSA59 infection show increased viral spread and decreased microglia/ macrophage activation. About 4–5-week-old Ifit2$^{-/-}$ mice upon RSA59 infection showed a robust viral replication and antigen spread throughout the brain parenchyma compared to the wildtype mice infection. Infectious viral load was significantly higher in the Ifit2$^{-/-}$ mice when assessed by plaque assay (A). The cryosections form Ifit2$^{-/-}$ and wildtype mice brain sections showed similar overall distribution of RSA59 but the total EGFP expression (viral antigen) was more in Ifit2$^{-/-}$ mice (A). At day 5 p.i. H&E staining for the sagittal sections of the whole brain form WT (B) and Ifit2$^{-/-}$ mice (I) showed much milder meningitis (J) and encephalitis characterized by perivascular cuffing (K) and microglial nodule (L) formation in the Ifit2$^{-/-}$ compared to WT (C–E) mice. Similarly activated microglia/macrophage were much less in the Ifit2$^{-/-}$ mice (M–O) compared to the WT (F–H) mice as seen in Iba1 immunostaining. (P) Brain section of Ifit2$^{-/-}$ mice showed heightened viral infection as evident by the profuse viral N protein immunostaining. Ifit2$^{-/-}$ mice however showed a comparatively decreased Iba1 immunostaining indicative of impaired activation of microglia/macrophages compared to the wildtype mice. Adapted form Das Sarma et al [30].

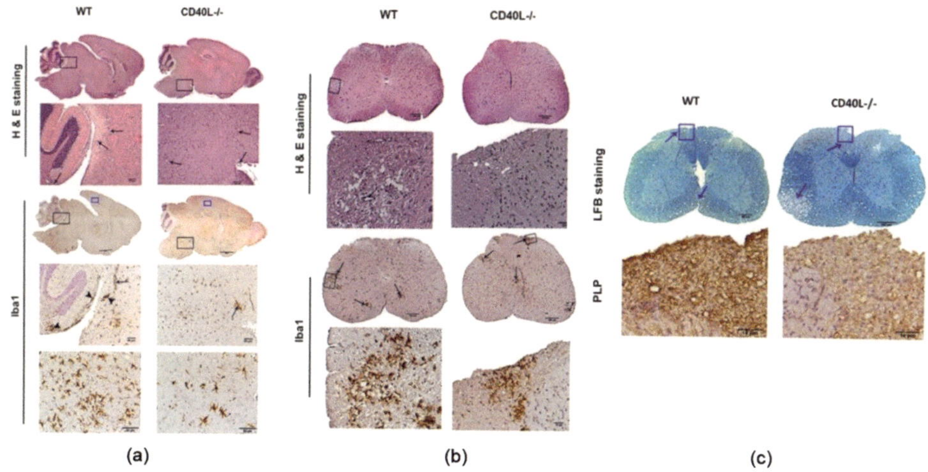

Figure 5.
RSA59 infection in CD40L deficient mice showed impaired microglia/macrophage activation during acute phase of neuroinflammation but causes profuse chronic demyelination concurrent with diminished PLP staining. (a and b) CD40L$^{-/-}$ and WT mice at day 5 upon RSA59 infection showed acute encephalitis and myelitis.Iba1 immunostaining in these brain and spinal cord sections showed that the CD40L$^{-/-}$ mice showed reduced Iba1+ cells compared to WT mice. (c) At day 30 p.i., spinal cord of CD40L$^{-/-}$ mice showed more intense demyelination and reduced PLP staining compared to wildtype mice. Adapted from Saadi et al [89].

impaired CD40-CD40L signaling in CD40L$^{-/-}$ mice, their priming is reduced substantially in the draining lymph nodes [89]. Effector CD4^{+} T cell population was reduced as well as the antiviral response was diminished, and phagocytic microglia persisted in the CNS at a substantial amount in the CD40L$^{-/-}$ mice. As a result, CD40L$^{-/-}$ mice exhibited greater demyelination, axonal loss, and persistent poliomyelitis at the chronic phase of infection [89]. Together, these studies highlight that migration of peripheral T cells and their interaction with microglia via CD40-CD40L is essential to eliminate the virus and provide long-term neuroprotection.

Independent of the effect on T cells, IFN produced by microglia acts on other cells that exert indirect antiviral effects [90]. For example, microglia induce antiviral functions in neurons via STING signaling and stimulate IFN-1 production in astrocytes by the TLR3 pathway [91]. Studies have shown that the Type 1 IFNAR signaling in astrocytes helps to protect the blood-brain barrier against virus infection and immunopathology [92]. Depletion of IFNAR signaling in astrocytes resulted in increased inflammatory cytokines and chemokines production, which caused blood-brain barrier inflammation during neurotropic viral infection [92].

Additionally, microglia also mediate viral clearance by autophagy [59]. Viral infections induce NFkB-dependent inflammatory effectors that produce antiviral molecules, including those promoting autophagy. ZIKV infection in Drosophila induces a stimulator of interferon genes (dSTING) in the brain, which promotes autophagy and helps protect the brain [93]. In mammals, autophagy has been shown to restrict HSV-1 infection [94]. Autophagy by microglia helps to clear the virus without causing cell death which protects mature neurons. Microglial phagocytosis is another mechanism that helps protect the neurons from severe damage. Microglia and neurons express C3aR that recognizes C3 cleavage products. In response to C3 and its cleavage products, microglia surround the neurons and phagocytose the presynaptic ends of the neurons [95]. This prevents the trans-synaptic spread of the virus and keeps neurons from firing abnormal signals that may result in cognitive impairment and physical disabilities.

Additionally, detrimental effects of microglia are also reported in many studies on viral encephalitis. Microglia are reported to remain persistently activated in several viral infections [80, 89]. Their activation is further associated with the production of TNF-α [96, 97], which can activate the astrocytic TNFR-1 pathway [98]. This signaling accentuates their crosstalk with neurons leading to modification of the excitatory synapses, which emerges in cognitive disabilities. TNF-α secreted by microglia can directly affect synaptic transmission and plasticity [62]. ZIKV infection has been associated with neurological damage among infants. Studies have found that ZIKV majorly infects the fetal microglia and activates them [61]. This induces an intense pro-inflammatory response by the secretion of mediators like IL-6, TNF-α, IL-1β, and MCP-1 [61]. Also, in HIV encephalitis, many microglia genes undergo significant changes, including immune activation and function, kinases, phosphatases, and pro-/anti-apoptotic and neurotrophic factors, which indicates that microglia functions are compromised and skewed towards pro-inflammation [99].

Thus, it can be ascertained that, microglia are not only important to maintain homeostasis in the CNS but are also critical for responding to injury, infection, and neurodegeneration. Often microglia act quickly in response to injury but with varied stimuli received, their activation profile can differ and may result in harmful or beneficial effects. It is true that viral encephalitis has caused high morbidity, which is a grave concern, but it is also imperative that research on microglia and viral encephalitis can provide new and efficient targets for treatment. Considering the unique response of microglia with different viral infections and at different stages of encephalitis, it is needless to say that the current research on microglia and viral encephalitis remains is at a nascent state. Depending on the type of encephalitis, careful fine-tuning of microglial activation has the potential to improve the therapeutic effect of encephalitis, its prognosis and also reduce the sequelae of encephalitis.

5. Encephalitis caused by several other neurotropic virus families

Many viruses from numerous virus families in different geographical areas can induce immediate or delayed neuropathological manifestations in humans and animals [18, 100]. Infection by neurotropic viruses and their resultant immune response has the potential to irreversibly disrupt the complex structural and functional dynamics of the central nervous system, frequently leaving the patient with a poor or fatal prognosis. The incidences of virus-induced CNS disorder are significantly higher than the damage caused by other pathogens.

Members of several virus families are known to be neurotropic, e.g., herpes family viruses, flaviviruses, paramyxoviruses, alphaviruses, bunyaviruses, orthomyxoviruses, arenaviruses, enteroviruses, rhabdoviruses, coronaviruses, and picornaviruses. Specifically, some of the viruses from these families are viruses like SARS-CoV, MERS-CoV, herpes simplex virus, poliovirus, West Nile virus (WNV), Chikungunya virus (CHIKV), Zika virus (ZIKV), Japanese encephalitis virus (JEV), La Crosse encephalitis (LACV), Epstein-Barr virus (EBV), measles, and mumps viruses, among many others [100, 101]. These viruses have been frequently associated with significant encephalitis, as well as meningitis and myelitis in the CNS. The clinical disease outcome of the CNS virus infection depends on several factors, like the host immune status, viral genomic constitution, and other environmental factors [100]. There is also evidence suggesting coronaviruses such as α-CoVs (NL63 and 229E) and the β-CoVs (OC43, HKU1) being positive-sense single-stranded, enveloped RNA viruses, can induce numerous neurological manifestations along with systemic inflammations in humans. A very recent outbreak of human β coronavirus SARS-CoV-2 is primarily known for its ARDS and paramount evidence suggest that it may enter the brain via olfactory route or can enter through the lung brain axis or gut-brain axis and is also known to cause meningitis, encephalitis, and demyelination [102–104].

The etiology of CNS infections induced by viruses can also depend on and vary across variable geographical locations. For example, reports have shown that herpes simplex viruses are the most common pathogens observed among both children and adults in the United States (US), Australia, and Italy. In contrast, in Southeast Asian countries like southern Vietnam, the Japanese encephalitis virus has been shown to be one of the most frequent inducers of viral encephalitis, especially among children. Enteroviruses have been commonly isolated to be involved in causing encephalitis in several parts of India. At the same time, HSVs have been observed to be more prevalent in the eastern parts of India, both among adults as well as children. Furthermore, the virulence of the viruses also varies geographically [105]. Therefore, understanding the etio-biology and epidemiology of neurotropic viruses is paramount in designing the targeted intervention.

Therefore, based on epidemiological prevalence and episodic occurrence evidence as well as the employment of these viruses as experimental model systems for human disorders, this book chapter will also briefly discuss some of the other viruses.

Flaviviruses are the enveloped, single-stranded, positive-sense RNA viruses that consist of the world's most clinically critical viruses like the following species: Japanese encephalitis virus (JEV), tick-borne encephalitis virus (TBEV), and Powassan encephalitis virus (POWV), as well as other mosquito-borne viruses, like Dengue virus (DENV), yellow fever virus (YFV), West Nile virus (WNV), St. Louis encephalitis virus (SLEV), and Zika virus (ZIKV) [106, 107]. JEV is highly prevalent in the Southeast Asian countries as well as the Indian subcontinent, affecting infants and children, and can also be transmitted to the fetus during pregnancy [108, 109]. The incidences of Tick-borne encephalitis (transmitted to humans by the bites of ticks) are progressively expanding in European and Asian countries with severe neurological complications [110]. WNV infection is endemic in temperate and tropical regions throughout the world, triggering yearly outbreaks of encephalitis [111]. St. Louis encephalitis virus (SLEV) is found predominantly in North, Central, and South America and accounts for nearly 35–60% of meningitis in all symptomatic cases in children [112, 113]. Zika virus is also an emerging pathogen with substantial clinical impact significantly on the CNS, as reported, in the form of severe congenital malformations (microcephaly) and neurological complications, mainly Guillain-Barré syndrome (GBS) [114]. It has shown explosive outbreaks in African, South, and Central American countries [112, 115].

Alphaviruses like Eastern equine encephalitis virus (EEEV), Western equine encephalitis virus (WEEV), and Venezuelan equine encephalitis virus (VEEV), as well as the Mayaro virus (MAYV), Una virus (UNAV), and Chikungunya virus (CHIKV) are the small, enveloped viruses with a single-stranded, positive-sense RNA [100, 113]. The most critical neurotropic alphavirus is VEEV, which induced many outbreaks in South, Central, and North America [116]. CHIKV has also caused severe neurological complications in humans at all age groups, especially in infants, in Europe, Asia, and Africa [117, 118]. EEEV can also induce encephalitis in humans in about 50–75% of the cases [8, 119].

Herpes family viruses which are double-stranded DNA viruses, have been commonly associated with severe encephalitis and meningitis in the CNS and have been distributed globally. The members of herpes family viruses that are shown to be neurotropic include HSV types 1 and 2, varicella-zoster, Epstein-Barr virus, and cytomegalovirus [120, 121]. Both children and immunocompromised individuals are most vulnerable to herpes simplex meningoencephalitis [120]. Another critical property to herpes family viruses, especially varicella-zoster virus, is reactivation [122]. Primary infection with VZV during childhood induces chickenpox, but the virus becomes latent in the spinal and cranial ganglia. However, deteriorating cellular immunity with senescence or immunocompromised conditions may lead to virus reactivation that promotes zoster (shingles) [123, 124].

Paramyxoviruses that induce neurological diseases are from genera Rubulavirus (consisting of the mumps virus), which is neurotropic [125]; Morbillivirus genera (consisting of measles virus) [126] and Henipavirus with the emerging Nipah virus (NiV) being one of the neurotropic variants [127]. These are single-stranded, nonsegmented RNA viruses [128]. Measles virus-induced encephalitis is one of the leading causes of morbidity and mortality in the developing world [129]. Nipah virus is one of the emerging viruses that present with numerous cases of acute encephalitis in humans [127, 130].

Lymphocytic choriomeningitis virus (LCMV) belonging to the family Arenaviridae is an enveloped, single-stranded RNA virus. Although its primary host is mice, it is also present in other rodents and has the ability to infect humans, especially laboratory workers, pet owners, and individuals living in impoverished conditions. It is predominant in Europe, Asia, American continents, and Africa [131–133].

Picornaviruses are single-stranded, non-enveloped RNA viruses encompassing enteroviruses (echoviruses, coxsackieviruses) and parechoviruses (PeVs) pathogenic against humans. Infants and children are highly susceptible to human pathogenic picornaviruses that induce aseptic meningitis and meningoencephalitis [134, 135]. It is highly predominant in the UK, Ireland, the US and some Southeast Asian countries [105, 136, 137].

6. Chronic viral encephalitis and neurodegeneration

The research on viral encephalitis is a rather dynamic and large field. However, its relationship with neurodegeneration is less explored. As research on viral encephalitis and neurodegenerative disease is progressing on diverse fronts many similarities are being identified between the classical neurodegenerative pathways and viral-induced neurodegeneration [138, 139]. It is well established that many neurotropic viruses result in neuronal dysfunction which can have devastating life threatening consequences for the host [138, 140, 141]. Virus can either directly infect the neurons and kill the cells directly by replication and lysis or by apoptosis as observed in poliomyelitis [139, 142]. Additionally viral-induced encephalitis can damage the neurons in an immune mechanism as all neurotropic virus infections irrespective of the route of entry can trigger both innate and adaptive immune responses [139, 143, 144]. Supporting this concept, a number of viruses have been associated with neurodegeneration outcomes [141]. For example, In addition to causing encephalitis, CMV infection can result in transverse myelitis [145], HIV is associated with severe dementia [146] and Echo virus can cause neuro-muscular disorder [147]. Additionally, yearlong infection with JEV in humans can cause postencephalitic parkinsonism (PEP) which shows symptoms similar to sporadic Parkinson's disease (PD) [148]. Evidence also suggests that H5N1 influenza virus induces many PD-like symptoms [149, 150].

Specifically, the virus first infects the peripheral nervous system (PNS) and later gains entry into the CNS where it causes degeneration of susceptible dopamine (DA) neurons in midbrain regions similar to PD patients [149, 151]. Another influenza virus strain H3N2 causes many neurodegenerative symptoms like amyotrophy, MS flares and relapsing delirium [152, 153]. However, the direct role of viruses in neurodegeneration is less understood. Most likely, several viruses have developed means to evade the immune response and are present in subclinical levels [154–156]. The local inflammatory response in the CNS in response to persistent virus infections results in chronic encephalomyelitis even without overt cell death which may lead to neuronal damage resulting in degeneration.

HSV-1 is one of the most common virus infections that can remain dormant in the neurons for life-long [157]. It is highly neurotropic and periodic reactivation is observed to establish productive infection of the neurons [140]. It is one of the largely associated viruses with Alzheimer's disease (AD) [158]. The virus presence is detected in the AD brains, in fact the presence of HSV-1 DNA on APOE gene carriers is a risk factor for AD [159]. Studies also showed HSV-1 DNA and amyloid β to be present in close proximity in AD plaques [160, 161]. Mechanistically, HSV-1 infection can promote neurotoxic Aβ accumulation, tau phosphorylation and cleavage as observed *in vitro* [161–163]. In addition to the direct interaction which the virus exploits to travel to the cell surface it also interferes with post-transcriptional regulation by up regulating microRNA-146a, which is another marker for AD [164].

Parkinson's disease (PD) the second most common neurodegenerative disorder has been linked to Influenza viruses [140, 165]. Highly neurotropic and pathogenic H5N1 virus can enter the CNS, induce encephalitis associated with microglial activation, loss of dopaminergic neurons and accumulation of α-synuclein aggregates in infected regions resembling PD symptoms and pathology [149, 166]. It is well documented that with the 1918 epidemic of H1N1 has greatly increased the incidence of PD [166]. Both H1N1 and H5N1 are found in the substantia nigra region which is also majorly affected in PD patients [167]. In fact, post-mortem brain sections from PD patients show the presence of influenza A virus [168]. No direct mechanism is yet established but is majorly thought to be a contribution of the neuroinflammation process activated by the virus in the CNS [151]. Moreover, HIV infection of the CNS is associated with amyotrophic lateral sclerosis (ALS), which is a fatal neurodegenerative disease with characteristic degeneration of the spinal cord and cortical neurons [169, 170]. Several other neurological symptoms are associated with HIV infections; the most common is HIV-associated dementia which shows certain complications presented with MS [171, 172]. HIV-associated dementia (HAD) also has many similarities with AD and PD including the target anatomical region hippocampus and substantia nigra [173]. The similarities of HAD with neurodegenerative disorders is reported at genomic, proteomic as well as transcription levels [140].

Modern times have seen a drastic increase in the average life expectancy which has come with its own limitation i.e., the incidence of ageing disorders. As discussed, virus infection can significantly act as co factors of neurodegeneration if not the causative agents. Also, the mechanism of viral and non-viral neurodegeneration is not very different [138, 140]. Both show an involvement of immune system by means of neuroinflammation and direct or indirect damage of neurons. Viruses can significantly modulate the structure and function of cytoskeletal proteins that are instrumental in neuronal dysfunction associated with neurodegeneration [174]. Thus, neurotropic virus infection for encephalitis and neuroinflammation can serve as excellent models for understanding neurodegeneration. Moreover, a better understanding of targeting the immune system, which has profound implications, especially in viral-induced neurodegeneration and deciphering the critical overlaps and distinctions between classical neurodegeneration and viral-induced neurodegeneration, can lead to developing new and efficient therapeutic strategies.

7. Conclusion

Encephalitis was considered a rare syndrome, but the incidence of encephalitis is likely to be elevated than previously estimated. This underrated approach towards understanding encephalitis prevails because it is challenging to diagnose, manage and study. Encephalitis is a condition with multiple etiologies and pathogeneses, ranging from direct infectious to immune-mediated; however, each of these specific mechanisms is diverse and often incompletely understood. Accurate diagnosis of encephalitis cases is made complicated because of the difficulties involved in distinguishing between encephalitic and non-encephalitis mimics, autoimmune vs. infectious encephalitis, and the limitation of standard clinical case/laboratory definitions. Ancillary testing, and clinical correlations, along with a clinical follow-up, are important to establish more specific diagnoses. Determining the etiology is the key first step to improving patient outcomes, and it needs advanced neuropathologic and clinical algorithms. Furthermore, the most recent antibody-associated forms of encephalitis also pose a challenge due to their significantly varying clinical manifestations. Understanding the antigenic specificity of intrathecal IgGs found in the CSF may help to identify clues to the cause of infection or inflammation in several cases of encephalitis.

Also, it is critical to study host-immune responses and other host factors to design novel therapeutic interventions, given the paradoxical role of the immune system in encephalitis. The increased urbanization, travel, and climate change are some of the factors, which contribute to the evolution and spread of new pathogens. Infectious diseases are emerging profoundly. Neuroinfectious diseases might occur as occurrences in small, localized regions or may rapidly spread over large geographical areas as pandemics, just like SARS-CoV2. Understanding emerging viruses need better experimental animal models, which will help to comprehend the cause-effect relationship between the virus and its associated neuropathogenesis. Strong consideration should be given to trials of combination therapy that include treatment strategies with both anti-inflammatory and anti-pathogen drugs.

Acknowledgements

Neurotopic m-CoV research in an experimental animal model has provided a timely and appropriate platform to take a step toward writing this comprehensive book chapter on encephalitis. This work has been a collaborative effort for two decades between the Indian Institute of Science Education and Research Kolkata (IISER-K), India; Indian Institute of Sciences (IISc), India; University of Pennsylvania, USA; Thomas Jefferson University, USA and University of Colorado Denver, USA. The joint endeavor has been supported and nurtured by the Indo-U.S. Science and Technology Forum (IUSSTF) on several occasions. m-CoV research was generously funded by the Department of Biotechnology (DBT), India, Council for Scientific and Industrial Research (CSIR), India; National Multiple Sclerosis

Society, USA; M.E. Groff Surgical Medical Research and Education Charitable Trust; and Lindback Foundation Career Enhancement Award, USA. The authors would also like to express their gratefulness to Dr. Dhriti Chatterjee, Dr. Kaushiki Biswas, Dr. Abhinoy Kishore, Dr. Subhajit Das Sarma, Dr. Afaq Hussain, Mr. Soumya Kundu, Mr. Abhishek Bose, Mr. Sourodip Sengupta, Ms. Mithila Kamble, Ms. Vaishali Mulchandani, Mr. Saurav, Mr. A. Safiriyu Abass, Dr. Mahua Maulik, and Ms. Soma Nag who have contributed immensely to the generation of a large volume of work on m-CoV research over the years. Authors would like to thank Dr. Kenneth S. Shindler, Dr. Lawrence C. Kenyon, and Dr. Randall J. Cohrs for their long-standing collaboration on m-CoV research. The success of this work has been primarily dependent on the collaborative efforts of the national and international m-COVID team and many researchers whose names are listed in the references.

Ethical statement

Most of the m-CoV work discussed in this chapter either adopted from our published work or from other studies adhered to the experimental procedures and animal care and use in accordance with good animal ethics approved by the Institutional Animal Care and use Committee.

Author details

Fareeha Saadi†, Debanjana Chakravarty†, Grishma Kasle† and Jayasri Das Sarma*
Department of Biological Sciences, Indian Institute of Science Education and Research Kolkata, Mohanpur, India

*Address all correspondence to: dassarmaj@iiserkol.ac.in

† These authors have contributed equally.

References

[1] Roos KL. Encephalitis. In: Handbook of Clinical Neurology. Vol. 121. Elsevier; 2014. pp. 1377-1381

[2] Granerod J, Ambrose HE, Davies NW, Clewley JP, Walsh AL, Morgan D, et al. Causes of encephalitis and differences in their clinical presentations in England: A multicentre, population-based prospective study. The Lancet Infectious Diseases. 2010;**10**(12):835-844

[3] Kennedy PGE. Viral encephalitis: Causes, differential diagnosis, and management. Journal of Neurology, Neurosurgery, and Psychiatry. 2004;**75**(Suppl. 1):i10-ii5

[4] Mace SE. Central nervous system infections as a cause of an altered mental status? What is the pathogen growing in your central nervous system? Emergency Medicine Clinics of North America. 2010;**28**(3):535-570

[5] Solomon T, Michael BD, Smith PE, Sanderson F, Davies NW, Hart IJ, et al. Management of suspected viral encephalitis in adults--Association of British Neurologists and British Infection Association National Guidelines. The Journal of Infection. 2012;**64**(4):347-373

[6] Kneen R, Michael BD, Menson E, Mehta B, Easton A, Hemingway C, et al. Management of suspected viral encephalitis in children—Association of British Neurologists and British Paediatric Allergy, Immunology and Infection Group national guidelines. The Journal of Infection. 2012;**64**(5):449-477

[7] Tunkel AR, Glaser CA, Bloch KC, Sejvar JJ, Marra CM, Roos KL, et al. The management of encephalitis: Clinical practice guidelines by the Infectious Diseases Society of America. Clinical Infectious Diseases: An Official Publication of the Infectious Diseases Society of America. 2008;**47**(3):303-327

[8] Whitley RJ. Viral encephalitis. New England Journal of Medicine. 1990;**323**(4):242-250

[9] Irani DN. Aseptic meningitis and viral myelitis. Neurologic Clinics. 2008;**26**(3):635-655

[10] Rotbart HA. Viral meningitis. Seminars in Neurology. 2000;**20**(03):277-292

[11] Kennedy PGE, Quan P-L, Lipkin WI. Viral encephalitis of unknown cause: Current perspective and recent advances. Viruses. 2017;**9**(6):138

[12] Venkatesan A, Murphy OC. Viral encephalitis. Neurologic Clinics. 2018;**36**(4):705-724

[13] Koyuncu OO, Hogue IB, Enquist LW. Virus infections in the nervous system. Cell Host & Microbe. 2013;**13**(4):379-393

[14] Ayala-Nunez NV, Gaudin R. A viral journey to the brain: Current considerations and future developments. PLoS Pathogens. 2020;**16**(5):e1008434

[15] Rozenberg F. Acute viral encephalitis. In: Handbook of Clinical Neurology. Vol. 112. Elsevier; 2013. pp. 1171-1181

[16] Chen Z, Zhong D, Li G. The role of microglia in viral encephalitis: A review. Journal of Neuroinflammation. 2019;**16**(1):76

[17] Tröscher AR, Wimmer I, Quemada-Garrido L, Köck U, Gessl D, Verberk SGS, et al. Microglial nodules provide the environment for pathogenic

T cells in human encephalitis. Acta Neuropathologica. 2019;**137**(4):619-635

[18] Chhatbar C, Prinz M. The roles of microglia in viral encephalitis: From sensome to therapeutic targeting. Cellular & Molecular Immunology. 2021;**18**(2):250-258

[19] Griffin DE, Metcalf T. Clearance of virus infection from the CNS. Current Opinion in Virology. 2011;**1**(3):216-221

[20] Das SJ. A mechanism of virus-induced demyelination. Interdisciplinary Perspectives on Infectious Diseases. 2010;**2010**:109239

[21] Saadi F, Pal D, Sarma JD. Spike Glycoprotein Is Central to Coronavirus Pathogenesis-Parallel Between m-CoV and SARS-CoV-2. Annals of Neurosciences. 2021. DOI: 10.1177/09727531211023755

[22] Lane TE, Buchmeier MJ. Murine coronavirus infection: A paradigm for virus-induced demyelinating disease. Trends in Microbiology. 1997;**5**(1):9-14

[23] Stohlman SA, Bergmann CC, Perlman S. In: Ahmed R, Chen I, editors. Persistent Viral Infections. New York: Wiley & Sons; 1998. pp. 537-557

[24] Buchmeier MJ, Lewicki HA, Talbot PJ, Knobler RL. Murine hepatitis virus-4 (strain JHM)-induced neurologic disease is modulated in vivo by monoclonal antibody. Virology. 1984;**132**(2):261-270

[25] Houtman JJ, Fleming JO. Dissociation of demyelination and viral clearance in congenitally immunodeficient mice infected with murine coronavirus JHM. Journal of Neurovirology. 1996;**2**(2):101-110

[26] Lavi E, Gilden DH, Highkin MK, Weiss SR. Persistence of mouse hepatitis virus A59 RNA in a slow virus demyelinating infection in mice as detected by in situ hybridization. Journal of Virology. 1984;**51**(2):563-566

[27] Lavi E, Gilden DH, Wroblewska Z, Rorke LB, Weiss SR. Experimental demyelination produced by the A59 strain of mouse hepatitis virus. Neurology. 1984;**34**(5):597-603

[28] Das Sarma J, Fu L, Hingley ST, Lavi E. Mouse hepatitis virus type-2 infection in mice: An experimental model system of acute meningitis and hepatitis. Experimental and Molecular Pathology. 2001;**71**(1):1-12

[29] Shindler KS, Kenyon LC, Dutt M, Hingley ST, Sarma JD. Experimental optic neuritis induced by a demyelinating strain of mouse hepatitis virus. Journal of Virology. 2008;**82**(17):8882-8886

[30] Das Sarma J, Burrows A, Rayman P, Hwang MH, Kundu S, Sharma N, et al. Ifit2 deficiency restricts microglial activation and leukocyte migration following murine coronavirus (m-CoV) CNS infection. PLoS Pathogens. 2020;**16**(11):e1009034

[31] Perlman S, Evans G, Afifi A. Effect of olfactory bulb ablation on spread of a neurotropic coronavirus into the mouse brain. The Journal of Experimental Medicine. 1990;**172**(4):1127-1132. DOI: 10.1084/jem.172.4.1127

[32] Lavi E, Gilden DH, Highkin MK, Weiss SR. The organ tropism of mouse hepatitis virus A59 in mice is dependent on dose and route of inoculation. Laboratory Animal Science. 1986;**36**(2):130-135

[33] Rout SS, Singh M, Shindler KS, Das SJ. One proline deletion in the fusion peptide of neurotropic mouse hepatitis virus (MHV) restricts retrograde axonal

transport and neurodegeneration. The Journal of Biological Chemistry. 2020;**295**(20):6926-6935. DOI: 10.1074/jbc.RA119.011918

[34] Das Sarma J, Scheen E, Seo SH, Koval M, Weiss SR. Enhanced green fluorescent protein expression may be used to monitor murine coronavirus spread in vitro and in the mouse central nervous system. Journal of Neurovirology. 2002;**8**(5):381-391

[35] Das Sarma J, Iacono K, Gard L, Marek R, Kenyon LC, Koval M, et al. Demyelinating and nondemyelinating strains of mouse hepatitis virus differ in their neural cell tropism. Journal of Virology. 2008;**82**(11):5519

[36] Kenyon LC, Biswas K, Shindler KS, et al. Gliopathy of Demyelinating and Non-Demyelinating Strains of Mouse Hepatitis Virus. Frontiers in Cellular Neuroscience. 2015;**9**:488. DOI: 10.3389/fncel.2015.00488

[37] Biswas K, Das SJ. Effect of microtubule disruption on neuronal spread and replication of demyelinating and nondemyelinating strains of mouse hepatitis virus *in vitro*. Journal of Virology. 2014;**88**(5):3043

[38] Das Sarma J, Kenyon LC, Hingley ST, Shindler KS. Mechanisms of primary axonal damage in a viral model of multiple sclerosis. The Journal of Neuroscience. 2009;**29**(33):10272

[39] Chatterjee D, Addya S, Khan RS, Kenyon LC, Choe A, Cohrs RJ, et al. Mouse hepatitis virus infection upregulates genes involved in innate immune responses. PLoS One. 2014;**9**(10):e111351

[40] Bergmann CC, Lane TE, Stohlman SA. Coronavirus infection of the central nervous system: Host-virus stand-off. Nature Reviews Microbiology. 2006;**4**(2):121-132

[41] Chakravarty D, Saadi F, Kundu S, Bose A, Khan R, Dine K, et al. CD4 deficiency causes poliomyelitis and axonal blebbing in murine coronavirus-induced neuroinflammation. Journal of virology. 2020;**94**(14):e00548-20. DOI: 10.1128/JVI.00548-20

[42] Biswas K, Chatterjee D, Addya S, Khan RS, Kenyon LC, Choe A, et al. Demyelinating strain of mouse hepatitis virus infection bridging innate and adaptive immune response in the induction of demyelination. Clinical Immunology. 2016;**170**:9-19

[43] Oleszak EL, Chang JR, Friedman H, Katsetos CD, Platsoucas CD. Theiler's virus infection: A model for multiple sclerosis. Clinical Microbiology Reviews. 2004;**17**(1):174-207

[44] Theiler M. Spontaneous encephalomyelitis of mice, a new virus disease. The Journal of Experimental Medicine. 1937;**65**(5):705-719

[45] Oleszak EL, Kuzmak J, Good RA, Platsoucas CD. Immunology of Theiler's murine encephalomyelitis virus infection. Immunologic Research. 1995;**14**(1):13-33

[46] Murray PD, Pavelko KD, Leibowitz J, Lin X, Rodriguez M. CD4(+) and CD8(+) T cells make discrete contributions to demyelination and neurologic disease in a viral model of multiple sclerosis. Journal of Virology. 1998;**72**(9):7320-7329

[47] Tsunoda I, Fujinami RS. TMEV and neuroantigens: Myelin genes and proteins, molecular mimicry, epitope spreading, and autoantibody-mediated remyelination. In: Lavi E, Constantinescu CS, editors.

Experimental Models of Multiple Sclerosis. Boston, MA: Springer US; 2005. pp. 593-616

[48] Drescher KM, Pease LR, Rodriguez M. Antiviral immune responses modulate the nature of central nervous system (CNS) disease in a murine model of multiple sclerosis. Immunological Reviews. 1997;**159**:177-193

[49] Tsunoda I, Kuang LQ, Fujinami RS. Induction of autoreactive CD8+ cytotoxic T cells during Theiler's murine encephalomyelitis virus infection: Implications for autoimmunity. Journal of Virology. 2002;**76**(24):12834-12844

[50] Oleszak EL, Hoffman BE, Chang JR, Zaczynska E, Gaughan J, Katsetos CD, et al. Apoptosis of infiltrating T cells in the central nervous system of mice infected with Theiler's murine encephalomyelitis virus. Virology. 2003;**315**(1):110-123

[51] Chang JR, Zaczynska E, Katsetos CD, Platsoucas CD, Oleszak EL. Differential expression of TGF-beta, IL-2, and other cytokines in the CNS of Theiler's murine encephalomyelitis virus-infected susceptible and resistant strains of mice. Virology. 2000;**278**(2):346-360

[52] Sato S, Reiner SL, Jensen MA, Roos RP. Central nervous system cytokine mRNA expression following Theiler's murine encephalomyelitis virus infection. Journal of Neuroimmunology. 1997;**76**(1-2):213-223

[53] Fontana A, Frei K, Bodmer S, Hofer E, Schreier MH, Palladino MA Jr, et al. Transforming growth factor-beta inhibits the generation of cytotoxic T cells in virus-infected mice. Journal of Immunology (Baltimore, Md: 1950). 1989;**143**(10):3230-3234

[54] Fekete R, Cserép C, Lénárt N, Tóth K, Orsolits B, Martinecz B, et al. Microglia control the spread of neurotropic virus infection via P2Y12 signalling and recruit monocytes through P2Y12-independent mechanisms. Acta Neuropathologica. 2018;**136**(3):461-482

[55] Drokhlyansky E, Göz Aytürk D, Soh TK, Chrenek R, O'Loughlin E, Madore C, et al. The brain parenchyma has a type I interferon response that can limit virus spread. Proceedings of the National Academy of Sciences. 2017;**114**(1):E95

[56] Liu Y, Gordesky-Gold B, Leney-Greene M, Weinbren NL, Tudor M, Cherry S. Inflammation-induced, STING-dependent autophagy restricts Zika virus infection in the Drosophila brain. Cell Host & Microbe. 2018;**24**(1):57-68.e3

[57] Moy RH, Gold B, Molleston JM, Schad V, Yanger K, Salzano MV, et al. Antiviral autophagy restricts Rift Valley fever virus infection and is conserved from flies to mammals. Immunity. 2014;**40**(1):51-65

[58] Moretti J, Roy S, Bozec D, Martinez J, Chapman JR, Ueberheide B, et al. STING senses microbial viability to orchestrate stress-mediated autophagy of the endoplasmic reticulum. Cell. 2017;**171**(4):809-23.e13

[59] Levine B, Mizushima N, Virgin HW. Autophagy in immunity and inflammation. Nature. 2011;**469**(7330):323-335

[60] Alirezaei M, Kiosses WB, Fox HS. Decreased neuronal autophagy in HIV dementia: A mechanism of indirect neurotoxicity. Autophagy. 2008;**4**(7):963-966

[61] Lum FM, Low DK, Fan Y, Tan JJ, Lee B, Chan JK, et al. Zika virus infects human fetal brain microglia and induces inflammation. Clinical Infectious

Diseases: An Official Publication of the Infectious Diseases Society of America. 2017;**64**(7):914-920

[62] Santello M, Bezzi P, Volterra A. TNFα controls glutamatergic gliotransmission in the hippocampal dentate gyrus. Neuron. 2011;**69**(5):988-1001

[63] Saylor D, Dickens AM, Sacktor N, Haughey N, Slusher B, Pletnikov M, et al. HIV-associated neurocognitive disorder--pathogenesis and prospects for treatment. Nature Reviews Neurology. 2016;**12**(4):234-248

[64] Persidsky Y, Gendelman HE. Mononuclear phagocyte immunity and the neuropathogenesis of HIV-1 infection. Journal of Leukocyte Biology. 2003;**74**(5):691-701

[65] Gras G, Kaul M. Molecular mechanisms of neuroinvasion by monocytes-macrophages in HIV-1 infection. Retrovirology. 2010;7(1):30

[66] Burdo TH, Lackner A, Williams KC. Monocyte/macrophages and their role in HIV neuropathogenesis. Immunological Reviews. 2013;**254**(1):102-113

[67] Williams KC, Hickey WF. Central nervous system damage, monocytes and macrophages, and neurological disorders in AIDS. Annual Review of Neuroscience. 2002;**25**:537-562

[68] Wallet C, De Rovere M, Van Assche J, Daouad F, De Wit S, Gautier V, et al. Microglial cells: The main HIV-1 reservoir in the brain. Frontiers in Cellular and Infection Microbiology. 2019;**9**(362). DOI: 10.3389/fcimb.2019.00362

[69] Micallef S, Galea R. CMV encephalitis in an immune-competent patient. BMJ Case Reports. 2018:bcr2018224740. DOI: 10.1136/bcr-2018-224740

[70] Arribas JR, Storch GA, Clifford DB, Tselis AC. Cytomegalovirus encephalitis. Annals of Internal Medicine. 1996;**125**(7):577-587

[71] Grassi MP, Clerici F, Perin C, D'Arminio Monforte A, Vago L, Borella M, et al. Microglial nodular encephalitis and ventriculoencephalitis due to cytomegalovirus infection in patients with AIDS: Two distinct clinical patterns. Clinical Infectious Diseases: An Official Publication of the Infectious Diseases Society of America. 1998;**27**(3):504-508

[72] Mlakar J, Korva M, Tul N, Popović M, Poljšak-Prijatelj M, Mraz J, et al. Zika virus associated with microcephaly. The New England Journal of Medicine. 2016;**374**(10):951-958

[73] Luo H, Winkelmann ER, Zhu S, Ru W, Mays E, Silvas JA, et al. Peli1 facilitates virus replication and promotes neuroinflammation during West Nile virus infection. The Journal of Clinical Investigation. 2018;**128**(11):4980-4991

[74] Town T, Jeng D, Alexopoulou L, Tan J, Flavell RA. Microglia recognize double-stranded RNA via TLR3. Journal of immunology (Baltimore, Md: 1950). 2006;**176**(6):3804-3812

[75] Seitz S, Clarke P, Tyler KL. Pharmacologic depletion of microglia increases viral load in the brain and enhances mortality in murine models of flavivirus-induced encephalitis. Journal of Virology. 2018;**92**(16):e00525-18. DOI: 10.1128/JVI.00525-18

[76] Chhatbar C, Detje CN, Grabski E, Borst K, Spanier J, Ghita L, et al. Type I interferon receptor signaling of neurons and astrocytes regulates microglia activation during viral encephalitis. Cell Reports. 2018;**25**(1):118-29.e4

[77] Wheeler DL, Sariol A, Meyerholz DK, Perlman S. Microglia are required for

protection against lethal coronavirus encephalitis in mice. The Journal of Clinical Investigation. 2018;**128**(3):931-943

[78] Mendez-Fernandez YV, Johnson AJ, Rodriguez M, Pease LR. Clearance of Theiler's virus infection depends on the ability to generate a CD8+ T cell response against a single immunodominant viral peptide. European Journal of Immunology. 2003;**33**(9):2501-2510

[79] Sitati EM, Diamond MS. CD4+ T-cell responses are required for clearance of West Nile virus from the central nervous system. Journal of Virology. 2006;**80**(24):12060-12069

[80] Chakravarty D, Saadi F, Kundu S, Bose A, Khan R, Dine K, et al. CD4 deficiency causes poliomyelitis and axonal blebbing in murine coronavirus-induced neuroinflammation. Journal of Virology. 2020;**94**(14):e00548-20. DOI: 10.1128/JVI.00548-20

[81] Stohlman Stephen A, Hinton David R, Parra B, Atkinson R, Bergmann CC. CD4 T cells contribute to virus control and pathology following central nervous system infection with neurotropic mouse hepatitis virus. Journal of Virology. 2008;**82**(5):2130-2139

[82] Ciurkiewicz M, Herder V, Beineke A. Beneficial and detrimental effects of regulatory T cells in neurotropic virus infections. International Journal of Molecular Sciences. 2020;**21**(5):1705. DOI: 10.3390/ijms21051705

[83] Omura S, Kawai E, Sato F, Martinez NE, Minagar A, Al-Kofahi M, et al. Theiler's virus-mediated immunopathology in the CNS and heart: Roles of organ-specific cytokine and lymphatic responses. Frontiers in Immunology. 2018;**9**:2870. DOI: 10.3389/fimmu.2018.02870

[84] Ciurkiewicz M, Herder V, Khan MA, Uhde AK, Teich R, Floess S, et al. Cytotoxic CD8(+) T cell ablation enhances the capacity of regulatory T cells to delay viral elimination in Theiler's murine encephalomyelitis. Brain Pathology (Zurich, Switzerland). 2018;**28**(3):349-368

[85] Wu GF, Dandekar AA, Pewe L, Perlman S. CD4 and CD8 T cells have redundant but not identical roles in virus-induced demyelination. Journal of Immunology (Baltimore, Md: 1950). 2000;**165**(4):2278-2286

[86] Chua MM, MacNamara KC, San Mateo L, Shen H, Weiss SR. Effects of an epitope-specific CD8+ T-cell response on murine coronavirus central nervous system disease: Protection from virus replication and antigen spread and selection of epitope escape mutants. Journal of Virology. 2004;**78**(3):1150-1159

[87] Ponomarev ED, Shriver LP, Dittel BN. CD40 expression by microglial cells is required for their completion of a two-step activation process during central nervous system autoimmune inflammation. Journal of Immunology (Baltimore, Md: 1950). 2006;**176**(3):1402-1410

[88] Chen K, Huang J, Gong W, Zhang L, Yu P, Wang JM. CD40/CD40L dyad in the inflammatory and immune responses in the central nervous system. Cellular & Molecular Immunology. 2006;**3**(3):163-169

[89] Saadi F, Chakravarty D, Kumar S, Kamble M, Saha B, Shindler KS, et al. CD40L protects against mouse hepatitis virus-induced neuroinflammatory demyelination. PLoS Pathogens. 2021;**17**(12):e1010059

[90] Perry AK, Chen G, Zheng D, Tang H, Cheng G. The host type I interferon

response to viral and bacterial infections. Cell Research. 2005;**15**(6):407-422

[91] Reinert LS, Lopušná K, Winther H, Sun C, Thomsen MK, Nandakumar R, et al. Sensing of HSV-1 by the cGAS-STING pathway in microglia orchestrates antiviral defence in the CNS. Nature Communications. 2016;7:13348

[92] Daniels BP, Holman DW, Cruz-Orengo L, Jujjavarapu H, Durrant DM, Klein RS. Viral pathogen-associated molecular patterns regulate blood-brain barrier integrity via competing innate cytokine signals. MBio. 2014;**5**(5):e01476-e01414

[93] Morris O, Liu X, Domingues C, Runchel C, Chai A, Basith S, et al. Signal integration by the iκb protein pickle shapes Drosophila innate host defense. Cell Host & Microbe. 2016;**20**(3):283-295

[94] Joubert PE, Werneke SW, de la Calle C, Guivel-Benhassine F, Giodini A, Peduto L, et al. Chikungunya virus-induced autophagy delays caspase-dependent cell death. The Journal of Experimental Medicine. 2012;**209**(5):1029-1047

[95] Vasek MJ, Garber C, Dorsey D, Durrant DM, Bollman B, Soung A, et al. A complement-microglial axis drives synapse loss during virus-induced memory impairment. Nature. 2016;**534**(7608):538-543

[96] Lokensgard JR, Hu S, Sheng W, van Oijen M, Cox D, Cheeran MC, et al. Robust expression of TNF-alpha, IL-1beta, RANTES, and IP-10 by human microglial cells during nonproductive infection with herpes simplex virus. Journal of Neurovirology. 2001;7(3):208-219

[97] Hanisch UK. Microglia as a source and target of cytokines. Glia. 2002;**40**(2):140-155

[98] Habbas S, Santello M, Becker D, Stubbe H, Zappia G, Liaudet N, et al. Neuroinflammatory TNFα impairs memory via astrocyte signaling. Cell. 2015;**163**(7):1730-1741

[99] Ginsberg SD, Alldred MJ, Gunnam SM, Schiroli C, Lee SH, Morgello S, et al. Expression profiling suggests microglial impairment in human immunodeficiency virus neuropathogenesis. Annals of Neurology. 2018;**83**(2):406-417

[100] Ludlow M, Kortekaas J, Herden C, Hoffmann B, Tappe D, Trebst C, et al. Neurotropic virus infections as the cause of immediate and delayed neuropathology. Acta Neuropathologica. 2016;**131**(2):159-184

[101] Hatanpaa KJ, Kim JH. Neuropathology of viral infections. In: Handbook of Clinical Neurology. Vol. 123. Elsevier; 2014. pp. 193-214

[102] Mao L, Wang M, Chen S, He Q, Chang J, Hong C, et al. Neurological manifestations of hospitalized patients with COVID-19 in Wuhan, China: A retrospective case series study. medRxiv. 2020;**77**(6):683-690. DOI: 10.1001/jamaneurol.2020.1127

[103] Koralnik IJ, Tyler KL. COVID-19: A global threat to the nervous system. Annals of Neurology. 2020;**88**(1):1-11

[104] Chakravarty D, Das SJ. Murine-beta-coronavirus-induced neuropathogenesis sheds light on CNS pathobiology of SARS-CoV2. Journal of Neurovirology. 2021;**27**(2):197-216

[105] Abdullahi AM, Sarmast ST, Singh R. Molecular biology and epidemiology of neurotropic viruses. Cureus. 2020;**12**(8):e9674

[106] Salimi H, Cain MD, Klein RS. Encephalitic arboviruses: Emergence,

clinical presentation, and neuropathogenesis. Neurotherapeutics. 2016;**13**(3):514-534

[107] Solomon T. Flavivirus encephalitis. The New England Journal of Medicine. 2004;**351**(4):370-378. DOI: 10.1056/NEJMra030476

[108] Zhang Y, Wang Z, Chen H, Chen Z, Tian Y. Antioxidants: Potential antiviral agents for Japanese encephalitis virus infection. International Journal of Infectious Diseases: IJID: Official Publication of the International Society for Infectious Diseases. 2014;**24**:30-36

[109] Upadhyay RK. Epidemiology, disease transmission and pathogenesis caused by JE virus: Its prevention and control. American Journal of Infectious Diseases and Microbiology. 2015;**3**(1):38-64

[110] Bogovic P, Strle F. Tick-borne encephalitis: A review of epidemiology, clinical characteristics, and management. World Journal of Clinical Cases. 2015;**3**(5):430-441

[111] Hernández-Triana LM, Jeffries CL, Mansfield KL, Carnell G, Fooks AR, Johnson N. Emergence of West Nile virus lineage 2 in Europe: A review on the introduction and spread of a mosquito-borne disease. Frontiers in Public Health. 2014;**2**:271. DOI: 10.3389/fpubh.2014.00271

[112] Higuera A, Ramírez JD. Molecular epidemiology of dengue, yellow fever, Zika and Chikungunya arboviruses: An update. Acta Tropica. 2019;**190**:99-111

[113] Go YY, Balasuriya UBR, Lee C-k. Zoonotic encephalitides caused by arboviruses: Transmission and epidemiology of alphaviruses and flaviviruses. Clinical and Experimental Vaccine Research. 2014;**3**(1):58-77

[114] Beckham JD, Pastula DM, Massey A, Tyler KL. Zika virus as an emerging global pathogen: Neurological complications of Zika virus. JAMA Neurology. 2016;**73**(7):875-879

[115] Thomas SJ, Endy TP, Rothman AL, Barrett AD. 155—Flaviviruses (dengue, yellow fever, Japanese encephalitis, West Nile encephalitis, St. Louis encephalitis, tick-borne encephalitis, Kyasanur Forest disease, Alkhurma hemorrhagic fever, Zika). In: Bennett JE, Dolin R, Blaser MJ, editors. Mandell, Douglas, and Bennett's Principles and Practice of Infectious Diseases. 8th ed. Philadelphia: W.B. Saunders; 2015. pp. 1881-903.e6

[116] Guzmán-Terán C, Calderón-Rangel A, Rodriguez-Morales A, Mattar S. Venezuelan equine encephalitis virus: The problem is not over for tropical America. Annals of Clinical Microbiology and Antimicrobials. 2020;**19**(1):19

[117] Mehta R, Gerardin P, de Brito CAA, Soares CN, Ferreira MLB, Solomon T. The neurological complications of chikungunya virus: A systematic review. Reviews in Medical Virology. 2018;**28**(3):e1978

[118] Gérardin P, Couderc T, Bintner M, Tournebize P, Renouil M, Lémant J, et al. Chikungunya virus–associated encephalitis. A cohort study on La Réunion Island, 2005-2009. 2016;**86**(1):94-102

[119] Carrera JP, Cucunubá ZM, Neira K, Lambert B, Pittí Y, Liscano J, et al. Endemic and epidemic human alphavirus infections in Eastern Panama: An analysis of population-based cross-sectional surveys. The American Journal of Tropical Medicine and Hygiene. 2020;**103**(6):2429-2437

[120] Meyding-Lamadé U, Strank C. Herpesvirus infections of the central nervous system in immunocompromised

patients. Therapeutic Advances in Neurological Disorders. 2012;**5**(5): 279-296

[121] Gilden DH, Mahalingam R, Cohrs RJ, Tyler KL. Herpesvirus infections of the nervous system. Nature Clinical Practice Neurology. 2007;**3**(2):82-94

[122] Duarte LF, Farías MA, Álvarez DM, Bueno SM, Riedel CA, González PA. Herpes simplex virus type 1 infection of the central nervous system: Insights into proposed interrelationships with neurodegenerative disorders. Frontiers in Cellular Neuroscience. 2019;**13**:46. DOI: 10.3389/fncel.2019.00046

[123] Gershon AA, Breuer J, Cohen JI, Cohrs RJ, Gershon MD, Gilden D, et al. Varicella zoster virus infection. Nature Reviews. Disease Primers. 2015;**1**:15016

[124] Kennedy PGE, Gershon AA. Clinical features of varicella-zoster virus infection. Viruses. 2018;**10**(11):609

[125] Rubin S, Eckhaus M, Rennick LJ, Bamford CG, Duprex WP. Molecular biology, pathogenesis and pathology of mumps virus. The Journal of Pathology. 2015;**235**(2):242-252. DOI: 10.1002/path.4445

[126] Fisher DL, Defres S, Solomon T. Measles-induced encephalitis. QJM: An International Journal of Medicine. 2015;**108**(3):177-182

[127] Hossain MJ, Gurley ES, Montgomery JM, Bell M, Carroll DS, Hsu VP, et al. Clinical presentation of nipah virus infection in Bangladesh. Clinical Infectious Diseases: An Official Publication of the Infectious Diseases Society of America. 2008;**46**(7):977-984

[128] Vries RD, Jong A, Verburgh RJ, Sauerhering L, Nierop GP, Binnendijk RS, et al. Human paramyxovirus infections induce T cells that cross-react with zoonotic henipaviruses. mBio. 2020;**11**(4):e00972-20. DOI: 10.1128/mBio.00972-20

[129] Ferren M, Horvat B, Mathieu C. Measles encephalitis: Towards new therapeutics. Viruses. 2019;**11**(11):1017

[130] Singh RK, Dhama K, Chakraborty S, Tiwari R, Natesan S, Khandia R, et al. Nipah virus: Epidemiology, pathology, immunobiology and advances in diagnosis, vaccine designing and control strategies—a comprehensive review. The Veterinary Quarterly. 2019;**39**(1):26-55

[131] Wilson MR, Peters CJ. Diseases of the central nervous system caused by lymphocytic choriomeningitis virus and other arenaviruses. In: Handbook of Clinical Neurology. Vol. 123. Elsevier; 2014. pp. 671-681

[132] Bonthius DJ. Lymphocytic choriomeningitis virus: An underrecognized cause of neurologic disease in the fetus, child, and adult. Seminars in Pediatric Neurology. 2012;**19**(3):89-95

[133] Dräger S, Marx A-F, Pigny F, Cherpillod P, Eisermann P, Sendi P, et al. Lymphocytic choriomeningitis virus meningitis after needlestick injury: A case report. Antimicrobial Resistance & Infection Control. 2019;**8**(1):77

[134] de Crom SCM, Rossen JWA, van Furth AM, Obihara CC. Enterovirus and parechovirus infection in children: A brief overview. European Journal of Pediatrics. 2016;**175**(8):1023-1029

[135] Baggen J, Thibaut HJ, Strating JRPM, van Kuppeveld FJM. The life cycle of non-polio enteroviruses and how to target it. Nature Reviews Microbiology. 2018;**16**(6):368-381

[136] Kadambari S, Braccio S, Ribeiro S, Allen DJ, Pebody R, Brown D, et al. Enterovirus and parechovirus meningitis in infants younger than 90 days old in the UK and Republic of Ireland: A British paediatric surveillance unit study. Archives of Disease in Childhood 2019;**104**(6):552-557. DOI: 10.1136/archdischild-2018-315643

[137] Dumaidi K, Al-Jawabreh A, Samarah F, Zraiqi A, Yaseen D. Genetic diversity of the enteroviruses detected from cerebrospinal fluid (CSF) samples of patients with suspected aseptic meningitis in northern West Bank, Palestine in 2017. PLoS One. 2018;**13**(12):e0202243

[138] Deleidi M, Isacson O. Viral and inflammatory triggers of neurodegenerative diseases. Science Translational Medicine. 2012;**4**(121):121ps3

[139] van den Pol AN. Viral infections in the developing and mature brain. Trends in Neurosciences. 2006;**29**(7):398-406

[140] Zhou L, Miranda-Saksena M, Saksena NK. Viruses and neurodegeneration. Virology Journal. 2013;**10**(1):172

[141] Berth SH, Leopold PL, Morfini GN. Virus-induced neuronal dysfunction and degeneration. Frontiers in Bioscience (Landmark Edition). 2009;**14**:5239-5259

[142] Wang T, Town T, Alexopoulou L, Anderson JF, Fikrig E, Flavell RA. Toll-like receptor 3 mediates West Nile virus entry into the brain causing lethal encephalitis. Nature Medicine. 2004;**10**(12):1366-1373

[143] Boulanger LM. Immune proteins in brain development and synaptic plasticity. Neuron. 2009;**64**(1):93-109

[144] Préhaud C, Mégret F, Lafage M, Lafon M. Virus infection switches TLR-3-positive human neurons to become strong producers of beta interferon. Journal of Virology. 2005;**79**(20):12893-12904

[145] Fux CA, Pfister S, Nohl F, Zimmerli S. Cytomegalovirus-associated acute transverse myelitis in immunocompetent adults. Clinical Microbiology and Infection. 2003;**9**(12):1187-1190

[146] Brew BJ, González-Scarano F. HIV-associated dementia: An inconvenient truth. Neurology. 2007;**68**(5):324-325

[147] Horta-Barbosa L, Fuccillo DA, Sever JL. Chronic viral infections of the central nervous system. Journal of the American Medical Association. 1971;**218**(8):1185-1188

[148] Shoji H, Watanabe M, Itoh S, Kuwahara H, Hattori F. Japanese encephalitis and parkinsonism. Journal of Neurology. 1993;**240**(1):59-60

[149] Jang H, Boltz D, Sturm-Ramirez K, Shepherd KR, Jiao Y, Webster R, et al. Highly pathogenic H5N1 influenza virus can enter the central nervous system and induce neuroinflammation and neurodegeneration. Proceedings of the National Academy of Sciences of the United States of America. 2009;**106**(33):14063-14068

[150] Jang H, Boltz D, McClaren J, Pani AK, Smeyne M, Korff A, et al. Inflammatory effects of highly pathogenic H5N1 influenza virus infection in the CNS of mice. The Journal of Neuroscience : The Official Journal of the Society for Neuroscience. 2012;**32**(5):1545-1559

[151] Rohn TT, Catlin LW. Immunolocalization of influenza A virus and markers of inflammation in the human Parkinson's disease brain. PLoS One. 2011;**6**(5):e20495

[152] Sulkava R, Rissanen A, Pyhälä R. Post-influenzal encephalitis during the influenza A outbreak in 1979/1980. Journal of Neurology, Neurosurgery, and Psychiatry. 1981;**44**(2):161-163

[153] Neurological complications of influenza. British Medical Journal. 1970;**1**(5691):248-249

[154] Nath A, Johnson TP. Mechanisms of viral persistence in the brain and therapeutic approaches. The FEBS Journal. 2021. Online ahead of Print. DOI: 10.1111/febs.15871

[155] Lafon M. Immune evasion, a critical strategy for rabies virus. Developments in Biologicals. 2008;**131**:413-419

[156] Xie X, Zeng J. Neuroimmune evasion of Zika virus to facilitate viral pathogenesis. Frontiers in Cellular and Infection Microbiology. 2021;**11**:662447. DOI: 10.3389/fcimb.2021.662447

[157] Whitley RJ. Herpesviruses. 4th ed. Galveston (TX): University of Texas Medical Branch at Galveston; 1996

[158] Letenneur L, Pérès K, Fleury H, Garrigue I, Barberger-Gateau P, Helmer C, et al. Seropositivity to herpes simplex virus antibodies and risk of Alzheimer's disease: A population-based cohort study. PLoS One. 2008;**3**(11):e3637

[159] Itzhaki RF, Wozniak MA. Herpes simplex virus type 1 in Alzheimer's disease: The enemy within. Journal of Alzheimer's Disease: JAD. 2008;**13**(4):393-405

[160] Denaro FJ, Staub P, Colmer J, Freed DM. Coexistence of Alzheimer disease neuropathology with herpes simplex encephalitis. Cellular and Molecular Biology (Noisy-le-Grand, France). 2003;**49**(8):1233-1240

[161] Wozniak MA, Mee AP, Itzhaki RF. Herpes simplex virus type 1 DNA is located within Alzheimer's disease amyloid plaques. The Journal of Pathology. 2009;**217**(1):131-138

[162] Santana S, Recuero M, Bullido MJ, Valdivieso F, Aldudo J. Herpes simplex virus type I induces the accumulation of intracellular β-amyloid in autophagic compartments and the inhibition of the non-amyloidogenic pathway in human neuroblastoma cells. Neurobiology of Aging. 2012;**33**(2):430.e19-430.e33

[163] Piacentini R, Civitelli L, Ripoli C, Marcocci ME, De Chiara G, Garaci E, et al. HSV-1 promotes Ca^{2+}–mediated APP phosphorylation and Aβ accumulation in rat cortical neurons. Neurobiology of Aging. 2011;**32**(12):2323.e13-2323.e26

[164] Hill JM, Zhao Y, Clement C, Neumann DM, Lukiw WJ. HSV-1 infection of human brain cells induces miRNA-146a and Alzheimer-type inflammatory signaling. Neuroreport. 2009;**20**(16):1500-1505

[165] Obeso JA, Rodríguez-Oroz MC, Benitez-Temino B, Blesa FJ, Guridi J, Marin C, et al. Functional organization of the basal ganglia: Therapeutic implications for Parkinson's disease. Movement Disorders: Official Journal of the Movement Disorder Society. 2008;**23**(Suppl. 3):S548-S559

[166] Hoffman LA, Vilensky JA. Encephalitis lethargica: 100 years after the epidemic. Brain. 2017;**140**(8):2246-2251

[167] Takahashi M, Yamada T, Nakajima S, Nakajima K, Yamamoto T, Okada H. The substantia nigra is a major target for neurovirulent influenza A virus. The Journal of Experimental Medicine. 1995;**181**(6):2161-2169

[168] Gamboa ET, Wolf A, Yahr MD, Harter DH, Duffy PE, Barden H, et al. Influenza virus antigen in postencephalitic parkinsonism brain. Detection by immunofluorescence. Archives of Neurology. 1974;**31**(4):228-232

[169] Verma A, Berger JR. ALS syndrome in patients with HIV-1 infection. Journal of the Neurological Sciences. 2006;**240**(1-2):59-64

[170] MacGowan DJ, Scelsa SN, Waldron M. An ALS-like syndrome with new HIV infection and complete response to antiretroviral therapy. Neurology. 2001;**57**(6):1094-1097

[171] Zhou L, Diefenbach E, Crossett B, Tran SL, Ng T, Rizos H, et al. First evidence of overlaps between HIV-associated dementia (HAD) and non-viral neurodegenerative diseases: Proteomic analysis of the frontal cortex from HIV+ patients with and without dementia. Molecular Neurodegeneration. 2010;**5**:27

[172] Maruszak H, Brew BJ, Giovannoni G, Gold J. Could antiretroviral drugs be effective in multiple sclerosis? A case report. European Journal of Neurology. 2011;**18**(9):e110-e111

[173] Brew BJ, Crowe SM, Landay A, Cysique LA, Guillemin G. Neurodegeneration and ageing in the HAART era. Journal of Neuroimmune Pharmacology : The Official Journal of the Society on NeuroImmune Pharmacology. 2009;**4**(2):163-174

[174] Zambrano Á, Solis L, Salvadores N, Cortés M, Lerchundi R, Otth C. Neuronal cytoskeletal dynamic modification and neurodegeneration induced by infection with herpes simplex virus type 1. Journal of Alzheimer's Disease. 2008;**14**:259-269

Chapter 7

Impairment of the Cardiovascular System during SARS-CoV-2 Infection

Cristina Tudoran, Mariana Tudoran, Voichita Elena Lazureanu, Adelina Raluca Marinescu, Dorin Novacescu and Talida Georgiana Cut

Abstract

Although the infection with the severe acute respiratory syndrome (SARS-CoV-2) virus affects primarily the respiratory system, it became evident from the very beginning that the coronavirus disease 2019 (COVID-19) is frequently associated with a large spectrum of cardiovascular involvements such as myocarditis/pericarditis, acute coronary syndrome, arrhythmias, or thromboembolic events, explained by a multitude of pathophysiological mechanisms. Individuals already suffering of significant cardiovascular diseases were more likely to be infected with the virus, had a worse evolution during COVID-19, with further deterioration of their basal condition and increased morbidity and mortality, but significant cardiac dysfunctions were diagnosed even in individuals without a history of heart diseases or being at low risk to develop such a pathology. Cardiovascular complications may occur anytime during the course of COVID-19, persisting even during recovery and, potentially, explaining many of the persisting symptoms included now in terms as subacute or long-COVID-19. It is now well accepted that in COVID-19, the occurrence of cardiovascular impairment represents a significant negative prognostic factor, immensely rising the burden of cardiovascular pathologies.

Keywords: COVID-19, inflammation, cytokine storm, myocardial injury, heart failure, thromboembolic events, arrhythmias

1. Introduction

Since the end of 2019, when the first cases were documented in Wuhan (China), the corona virus disease 2019 (COVID-19), a zoonotic infection caused by the severe acute respiratory syndrome coronavirus 2 (SARS-CoV-2), has spread rapidly and rampantly, raising major concerns regarding public health, while applying an unprecedented, continuous strain, on the global medical infrastructure. COVID-19 was officially declared a pandemic by the World Health Organization on 11 March 2020 [1], and since then it has affected over 400 million people worldwide, with a cumulative mortality rate of under 2% [2] and recent alleviation of clinical outcomes due to the development and widespread implementation of efficient vaccination. Taking into account the extreme polymorphism of clinical presentations, ranging from asymptomatic to severe systemic effects, mainly involving the respiratory and cardiovascular systems, and fatal, rapidly progressing, acute respiratory distress syndrome (ARDS), the containment of transmission, at least in the pre-vaccination era, and the therapeutic management of COVID-19 and its systemic complications, has proven to be quite a challenge for clinicians, especially in the case of high-risk patients [3].

A novel member of the β-coronavirus genus, group 2, the enveloped, positive-sense RNA single-stranded SARS-CoV-2, has established itself as the third emerging, highly pathogenic coronavirus, to infect humans and cause a large-scale outbreak since the early 2000s, after severe acute respiratory syndrome coronavirus (SARS-CoV) and Middle East respiratory syndrome coronavirus (MERS-CoV) [4]. Even though mortality rates are lower for SARS-CoV2 than for previous related coronavirus outbreaks (>35% for MERS-CoV and > 10% for SARS-CoV), contagiousness is much higher (MERS-CoV and SARS-CoV had only 10000 cumulative cases between them), as transmission is mainly airborne (via respiratory droplets), with multiple alternative mechanisms being reported (aerosols, direct contact with contaminated surfaces, and fecal-oral transmission [4]).

From a genomic viewpoint, SARS-CoV-2 shares ~80% sequence identity with SARS-CoV and ~ 50% with MERS-CoV, encoding 16 nonstructural proteins (that make up the replicase complex), 9 accessory proteins, and 4 structural proteins – spike (S), envelope (E), membrane (M), and nucleocapsid (N). The SARS-CoV-2 life cycle revolves around the envelope S protein. Direct contact between the Spike receptor-binding domain and the innate cellular receptor (angiotensin-converting enzyme 2 – ACE2), if provided adequate cleavage of the viral Spike S1/S2 polybasic cleavage site by host-cell proteolytic enzymes, will ensure Spike activation in endosomes and virus-cell membrane fusion (cell surface and endosomal compartments), allowing viral RNA to be released into the host-cell cytosol. Viral replication ensues, with subsequent expulsion into the intercellular space [4]. In fact, the S gene of SARS-CoV-2 represents the distinguishing genomic feature from SARS-CoV, sharing <75% nucleotide identity [4].

The main tissue tropism of SARS-CoV-2 is pulmonary, targeting high ACE2 expression cells (airway/alveolar epithelial cells, vascular endothelial cells, and alveolar macrophages) [5]. Even so, higher levels of ACE2 messenger RNA expression can be found in many extra-pulmonary tissues as well and nearly undetectable amounts of ACE2 still support viral host-cell entry. Therefore, additional, underappreciated, cell-intrinsic factors must also be involved in host-cell entry [4]. Noteworthy, a subpopulation of human type II alveolar cells has been documented, which manifest abundant ACE2 expression, and concomitant high levels of messenger RNA, specific to certain cellular proviral genes (coding elements of the, SARS-CoV-2 cell entry facilitating, and endosomal transport system) [6]. Also, ACE2 expression regulation must be considered, as, during viral infection, ACE2 gene expression in human airway epithelial cells is upregulated by type I and II interferons [5].

Considering the multitude of the medical literature written on the topic of multisystem impairment occurred during the infection with the SARS-CoV-2 virus, the purpose of our research was to summarize the opinions of experts concerning the cardiovascular alterations associated with COVID-19, and for this aim we reviewed the most significant articles published on PubMed, Medline, and Research gate on these topics and provided individualized summaries of expert opinions.

2. Effects of the SARS-CoV-2 virus on the cardiovascular system

The COVID-19 pandemic greatly challenged clinicians, both due to the sheer number of patients, but also because of the lack of therapeutic consensus and incomplete understanding of disease pathogenesis. Most fatal cases of COVID-19 relate to a severe atypical pneumonia, accompanied by a sudden systemic deterioration, despite therapeutic intervention in the hospital setting.

The infection with the SARS-CoV-2 virus primarily affects the respiratory structures, but the involvement of the cardiovascular system is also frequent. Cardiovascular complications in addition to respiratory disease may develop in all phases of COVID-19, which can start with the dramatic picture of acute heart failure (ACF), acute coronary syndrome (ACS), pulmonary venous thromboembolism (VTE), or even sudden cardiac death, as shown in **Figure 1**. The pathophysiological mechanisms underlying these disproportionate effects of the SARS-CoV-2 infection on patients with cardiovascular comorbidities, however, remain incompletely understood [7]. Thromboembolic events, usually accompanied by violent, pulmonary, and/or systemic complications, have been described from early on, since the beginning of the pandemic, with infectious inflammatory response patterns rapidly shifting into a typical systemic inflammatory response syndrome (SIRS) or ARDS, which could potentially induce multi-organ failure (MOF) and, subsequently, death. As we enter the third year of the pandemic, COVID-19 pathophysiology is slowly unraveling as we begin to better comprehend the complex interplay between the direct cytotoxic effects of SARS-CoV-2 on pneumocytes and endothelial cells, the emerging local and systemic inflammatory response, and the ways in which these responses interact with hemostatic homeostasis, a mechanism which has been deemed as central and, at least to this extent, unprecedented [8].

2.1 Cardiac tissue damage

COVID-19 was initially considered to be solely a respiratory disease, yet clinical outcomes quickly revealed that, undeniably, this infection implies multi-organ involvement. Perhaps most notably, the heart has been shown to represents a target organ for SARS-CoV-2-related pathogenesis, with a high prevalence of cardiac injury following COVID-19, often diagnosed only through biomarker evaluation. Beyond subclinical myocardial damage, SARS-CoV-2 infection may also cause more aggressive, clinically apparent modifications, such as myocarditis, accompanied by a subsequent diastolic dysfunction or severe reduction of left ventricle ejection fraction, not to mention the fact that heart failure may represent a short–/long-term consequence of COVID-19-related inflammatory cardiomyopathy, with dramatic consequences regarding prognosis [9].

Regarding myocardial damage in COVID-19, although the full pathophysiology is still incompletely understood, multiple mechanisms are most likely incriminated (see **Figure 2**), which, globally, can be divided into two main groups: direct, specific modifications, related to the cytopathic effects of SARS-CoV-2 infection, and indirect, general modifications, commonly seen in other severe infections, as well [10].

2.1.1 Direct cytopathic myocardial injury

The aforementioned ACE2, a type I transmembrane protein, highly expressed in different organs (heart, lungs, gut, and kidneys), mediates SARS-CoV-2 entry into

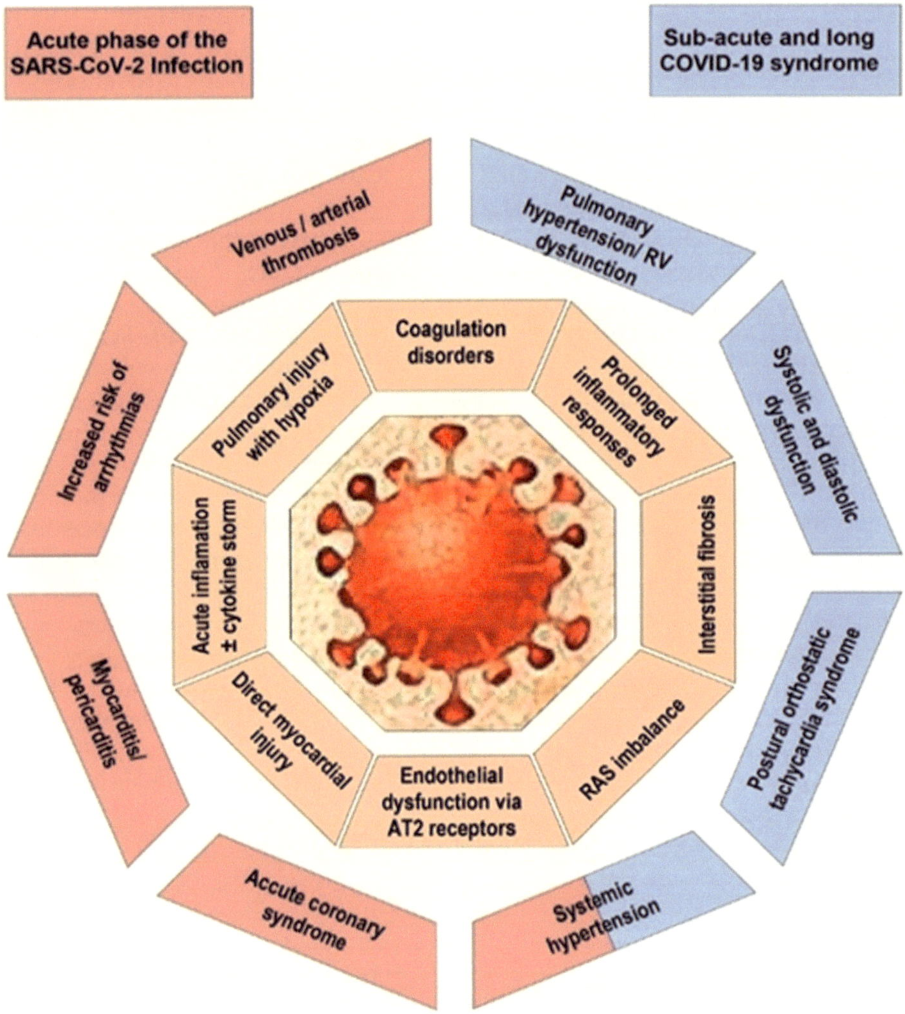

Figure 1.
Main COVID-19-associated cardiovascular complications and underlying pathophysiological mechanisms.

the host cells, with different clinical implications, depending on the targeted organ, and represents the key molecular entity involved in the direct cytopathic effects of SARS-CoV-2 infection within the cardiac tissue. After entering the host cell through the host ACE2 receptor, SARS-CoV-2 utilizes the host's RNA-dependent RNA polymerase to replicate its own structural proteins, which are then assembled, and the newly formed virions are released from the infected cells, perpetuating the viral life cycle. Theoretically, as a consequence of this process, infected cells may become damaged/destroyed [11].

This idea is supported by a recent autopsy study, analyzing cardiac tissue from 39 consecutive patients who died as a consequence of COVID-19, which found viral genome in the myocardial tissue, yet in situ hybridization showed that the most likely localization of SARS-CoV-2 not to be in the cardiomyocytes, but rather in interstitial cells or macrophages invading the myocardial tissue [12]. Even so, in engineered heart tissue models of COVID-19 myocardial pathology, SARS-CoV-2 demonstrated

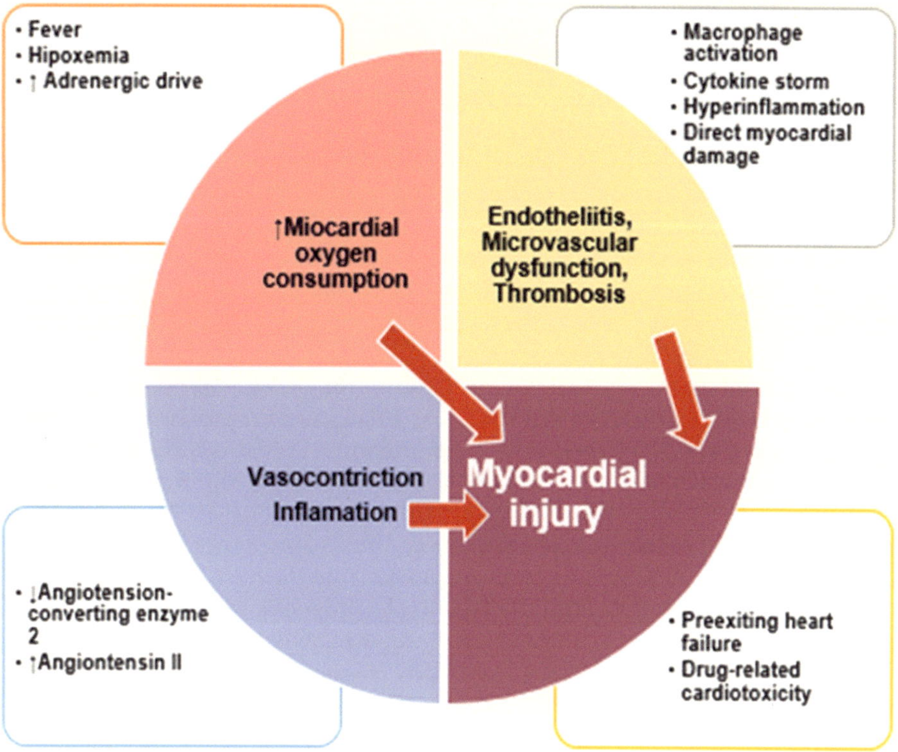

Figure 2.
Pathophysiology of COVID-19-related myocardial injury [15, 16].

the ability to directly infect cardiomyocytes through ACE2, resulting in contractile deficits, cytokine production, sarcomere disassembly, and cell death [9].

Furthermore, ACE2 must not be viewed as a mere bystander in the pathophysiology of COVID-19 myocardial injury, seeing as, besides being the host cell receptor of SARS-CoV-2, ACE2 is an enzyme involved in the renin-angiotensin-aldosterone system (RAAS). Specifically, ACE2 cleaves angiotensin II, a very potent vasoconstrictor, into angiotensin 1–7, which manifests vasodilator and anti-inflammatory effects. ACE2 also demonstrates a weak affinity for angiotensin I (or proangiotensin, formed by the action of renin on angiotensinogen), competitively limiting angiotensin II synthesis by ACE. Angiotensin I is converted by ACE2 into the nonapeptide angiotensin 1–9, which will manifest vasodilator effects through subsequent angiotensin type 2 (AT2) receptor stimulation. Therefore, ACE2 can counteract the undesirable effects of angiotensin II, demonstrating vasodilator, antioxidant, and anti-fibrotic effects [13]. In the context of SARS-CoV-2 infection, after S protein binding is complete, the virus attaches ACE2 through membrane fusion and invagination, causing a downregulation of ACE2 enzymatic activity [13]. Additionally, ACE2 also demonstrates immunomodulatory properties, both directly, via its interactions with macrophages, and indirectly, as it reduces expression of angiotensin II, which stimulates inflammation [14]. Thus, ACE2 downregulation in the context of SARS-CoV-2 infection may increase angiotensin II levels, favoring AT1 receptor activity, with a subsequent vasoconstriction, fibrotic, proliferative, and pro-inflammatory effects [10].

2.1.2 Indirect mechanisms of myocardial injury

As is the case with all severe respiratory infections, COVID-19 has a general deleterious effect on the cardiovascular system, with fever and sympathetic activation causing tachycardia and implicitly increasing myocardial oxygen consumption [9, 10], while prolonged bed rest and systemic inflammation will favor coagulation disorders, as supported by clinical findings – both venous and atypical arterial thromboembolic events have been documented in COVID-19 patients (see subchapter 3.4. Thromboembolic events and bleeding risk). Hypoxemia, another hallmark of COVID-19, will determine enhanced oxidative stress and increased production of reactive oxygen species, with subsequent intracellular acidosis, mitochondrial damage, and cell death [7, 9].

Moreover, another series of indirect mechanisms for COVID-19-related myocardial damage appears as a result of the abnormal inflammatory response which may be elicited by SARS-CoV-2 infection (i.e. a pro-inflammatory surge, the so-called "cytokine storm," which may occur as early as 1 week after the initial exposure and infection) [15].

Indeed, individual immune response is the cardinal element behind SARS-CoV-2 infection progression. Upon viral genome expulsion into the host cytosol, SARS-CoV-2 viral replication begins, with aberrant RNA sequences, byproducts of replication, being, in turn, detected by intracellular receptors, which activate the cellular antiviral response, involving enhanced leukocyte chemotaxis and transcriptional induction of type I and III interferons (IFN-I/-III), followed by under-regulation of IFN-stimulated genes [16]. Lung cell damage incurred during replication will also activate the local immune response, resulting in monocyte/macrophage recruitment [16], while chemokines will induce specific leukocyte subset recruitment and coordination [16]. Circulating immune cell relocation in the pulmonary tissue will determine additional cytokine/chemokine production, while also creating multiple imbalances in immune cell populations – increased leukocyte count and neutrophil-lymphocyte ratio, with decreased lymphocytes (especially T cells [17]), thus setting the scene for immune response dysregulation [3].

In fact, the relationship between SARS-CoV-2 infection and extensive activation of inflammation signaling pathways has been well documented, representing the main immunopathological mechanism through which severe forms occur, in susceptible individuals. During the acute phase of the infection, a disproportionate response occurs between T helper cell populations (types 1 and 2), characterized by high circulating levels of interleukin (IL)-1β, IL-1RA, IL-2, IL-6, IL-7, IL-8, IL-9 IL-10, interferon gamma-induced protein-10 (CXCL10), monocyte chemoattractant protein-1 (CCL2), macrophage inflammatory protein 1α (CCL3) and 1β (CCL4), granulocyte colony-stimulating factor, vascular endothelial growth factor (VEGF), and tumor necrosis factor (TNF) α [16, 18, 19], which mediate widespread lung inflammation, in an attempt to eradicate the pathogen [3]. The resulting hyper-inflammatory status, as well as the individual excessive levels of certain circulating cytokine species, have been independently associated with an unfavorable evolution and increased mortality [20]. This hyper-inflammatory state seems, at least intuitively, to be pivotal in the development of cardiac injury, seeing as positive correlations have been established between the increase in inflammatory markers and myocardial damage in COVID-19 [21, 22]. Indeed, this idea is additionally supported by previous studies, in other septic conditions, evidencing that the release of pro-inflammatory cytokines such as TNFα and IL-1β, were responsible for myocardial cells depression through modulation of calcium channel activity and nitric oxide production [23].

It may also be the case that the cytokine storm following SARS-CoV-2 infection determines the AHF, recurrently seen in severe COVID-19, as the inflammatory activation and oxidative stress background are similarly expressed generally in heart failure, predisposing to a more severe clinical course [24].

Lastly, the aforementioned marked inflammatory changes will also take place in the endothelium, as shown in postmortem histological studies, evidencing lymphocytic endotheliitis with apoptotic bodies and viral inclusion in multiple organs [7, 25]. Endotheliitis can lead to disseminated intravascular coagulation, with small or large vessels thrombosis and infarction, and will determine significant new vessel growth through a mechanism of intussusceptive angiogenesis [25].

2.2 Coagulation disturbances

After becoming infected, roughly 20% of COVID-19 patients will be incapable of controlling/halting viral replication through their initial immune response, which may be aberrant/insufficient or overwhelmed by a high initial viral load, or both [26]. This subgroup of patients will thus progress to a more severe disease phenotype, with aggravating symptomatology secondary to uncontrolled viral replication, leading to host pneumocyte and endothelial cell apoptosis, which in turn will activate platelets, induce procoagulant factor expression (fibrinogen, factors V, VII, VIII, X, and von Willebrand), and increase inflammatory response, as the body tries and fails to keep the infection localized to the lungs [27]. This sequence of host responses will additionally damage the pulmonary parenchyma (through further destruction of pneumocytes, microangiopathy, and inflammatory microthrombi), causing even more severe symptoms and hindering oxygenation, thus imposing the need for an additional oxygen supply. Even so, at this point, a relative balance between procoagulant and anticoagulant (but also pro-inflammatory/anti-inflammatory) factors is still maintained. In only approximately 5% of symptomatic patients, the pro-inflammatory processes involved in the immune response to SARS-CoV-2 infection will derail into the so-called "cytokine storm," which will fuel pro-inflammatory and pro-coagulatory processes even further, resulting in systemic endotheliitis and capillary leakage, cellular dysfunction, organ dysfunction (including ARDS), and overt activation of the (systemic) coagulation cascade resulting in the need for critical organ support [28]. In fact, SARS-CoV-2 infection may trigger endothelial dysfunction not only through the direct cytopathic effect of invasion on vascular endothelial cells but also through indirect mechanisms, such as hypoxia and the induced inflammatory response [27]. Moreover, some patients have also manifested antiphospholipid antibodies [28].

Therefore, all factors of the classic Virchow triad are influenced during the course of COVID-19, and they contribute synergically to the risk of thromboembolic events: hemodynamic changes (increased blood viscosity due to elevated fibrinogen, but also venous stasis due to hospitalization and disease-related immobilization); hypercoagulability (due to an overwhelming inflammatory state, occurring early after infection); and endothelial injury/dysfunction (ACE2 receptor expression on endothelial cells allows viral entry and cytopathic effects – endotheliitis) [3].

3. Acute cardiovascular complications of COVID-19

3.1 Myocarditis/pericarditis

It is generally accepted that viral infections, and corona viruses even more, are a common cause of myocarditis, frequently associated with congestive heart failure (CHF), and an increased risk to sudden death due to ventricular arrhythmias [29]. Emerging data suggest an increased association between myocarditis and COVID-19, observed more frequently in hospitalized patients, associated with an increased risk of adverse outcome, including higher mortality rates [30].

According to Dallas criteria, acute myocarditis is defined as "inflammatory infiltrate of the myocardium with necrosis and/or degeneration of adjacent myocytes not typical for the ischemic damage associated with coronary artery disease." Proposed pathophysiological pathways are myocardial injury due to the direct action of the virus, mediated via ACE2 receptors, and an intense, prolonged inflammatory response resulting in the release of high amounts of cytokines [29, 31, 32] together with additional factors such as hypoxia, increased metabolic demands, and physiological stress. At biopsy, myocyte and interstitial cells necrosis and mononuclear cell infiltrates were detected.

The real prevalence of acute myocarditis in patients infected with the SARS-CoV-2 virus is difficult to establish. In the medical literature, in these patients, the estimated incidence of acute myocarditis ranges from 12–17% or even 22–31% in ICU patients [33]. The symptoms vary from mild, nonspecific ones: palpitations, breathlessness, chest pain, common in influenza, to the dramatic picture of AHF with dyspnea, arrhythmias, or even sudden cardiac death. On the electrocardiogram (ECG), there are nonspecific ST, PR, and T-wave abnormalities, but signs mimicking an ACS, tachyarrhythmias, and conduction disturbances associated or not with left ventricular echocardiographic alterations and elevated levels of high sensitive troponins are also frequently seen [31, 33]. Another aspect is that the main diagnostic criteria require endomyocardial biopsy and cardiac magnetic resonance imaging (MRI), which are sometimes difficult or even impossible to access in COVID-19 patients due to the increased risk of contamination [33, 34]. It has been discussed that the prevalence of myocarditis rose parallel with the evolving strains of the SARS-CoV-2 virus being higher in patients infected in 2021 than in 2020 [30].

The incidence of pericarditis in COVID-19 patients ranges from 3% to 4.8% [35, 36]. It is often associated with myocarditis in COVID-19 patients with pneumonia and elevated inflammatory markers, as demonstrated by Diaz et al. in a meta-analysis performed on 33 studies, mainly case reports. The principal mechanism seems to be an autoreactive, inflammatory response [36].

Pericarditis manifests itself with a variety of symptoms, such as chest pain, fever, and dyspnea [36]. Pericardial friction rub is seldom encountered (9.3%) [36]. The predominant characteristic of this type of pericarditis is pericardial thickening observed at transthoracic echocardiography (TTE) persisting several weeks during recovery [37]. Over 50% of patients have pericardial effusion, mostly small to moderate in size, with 34% having large pericardial effusion, and even pericardial tamponade developed in about half of this last subset of patients [36]. On the ECG, 60% of patients present the typical four-stage evolution: diffuse ST elevation with depression of the PR segment, normalization of ST elevation, diffuse T-wave inversion, and in the end, normalization of the ECG [66]. Some patients presented unspecific signs, such as diffuse ST elevation, PR depression, and focal T-wave inversion [36].

The treatment of acute pericarditis consists in high doses of nonsteroidal anti-inflammatory drugs (NSAIDs) such as Ibuprofen, Indomethacin, or Naproxen recommended until symptom relief is achieved, and in addition, colchicine is recommended to be used for 3 to 6 months. Aspirin may be an alternative to NSAIDs [36]. Although low to moderate doses of steroids could be recommended in patients with SARS-CoV-2 infection, in most cases, this therapy is started sooner because of the associated viral myocarditis [36]. Furthermore, steroids can also be added to NSAIDs and colchicine as triple therapy for patients with an incomplete response. In the case of cardiac tamponade, pericardial drainage represents the standard of care [36]. Usually, the evolution of pericarditis associated with COVID-19 is benign.

3.2 Acute coronary syndrome

An increased incidence of ACS has been reported in several viral infections such as influenza, SARS, and MERS, being associated with a 3- to 10-fold increased risk, but in COVID-19 exact data are lacking [31, 32]. As principal potential pathophysiological pathways are considered: destabilization of atherosclerotic plaques due to systemic inflammation with an increased release of pro-inflammatory cytokines, the "cytokine storm," associated microangiopathy, activation of prothrombotic factors, as well as other specific changes of immune cell polarization toward more unstable phenotypes. Contributing factors also are myocardial oxygen supply/demand mismatch in the context of increased metabolic demands due to tachycardia/arrhythmias, fever, and hypoxia. These factors probably represent also the best explanation for the increased troponin levels observed in many patients with acute COVID-19 in the absence of typical cardiovascular manifestations (chest pain, specific ischemic electrocardiographic modification, and parietal hypokinesia at TTE) [31, 32], the more so as some other complications such as myopericarditis may have similar symptoms, and often patients with COVID-19 may not have typical angina symptoms.

Patients already suffering with coronary artery disease and heart failure may be exposed in a greater extent to ACS as a consequence of coronary plaque rupture or stent thrombosis in the context of systemic inflammation [31, 32]. For this reason, it is strongly recommended that in patients with a previous history of coronary artery disease and especially in those with coronary interventions, antiplatelet therapy should be continued, eventually even intensified, together with other plaque stabilizing agents such as statins, beta-blockers, and angiotensin-converting enzyme inhibitors [27, 30, 38, 39].

In this global health systems crisis, an adequate diagnosis and management of ACS is complicate and health care institutions worldwide have reexamined their protocols considering the increased risk of contamination of healthcare personal and the high requirements for protective equipment [34, 40, 41]. However, risk stratification is difficult due to limited bedside approach for an accurate ECG and TTE examination [31, 42]. The treatment of acute myocardial infarction (AMI) in COVID-19 patients is even more controversial. While in patients diagnosed with non-ST elevation myocardial infarction (non-STEMI), the result of a PCR testing could be expected prior to cardiac catheterization, in cases with ST elevation myocardial infarction (STEMI), the American College of Cardiology (ACC) recommends reconsidering fibrinolysis in patients with "low-risk STEMI" such as inferior without right ventricular extension, or lateral STEMI without altered hemodynamic. Thus percutaneous coronary intervention (PCI) remains the most indicated therapy, remaining the best option also in non-STEMI patients who are hemodynamically unstable [34, 42, 43].

In a large meta-analysis, DeLuca et al. concluded that COVID-19 pandemic has significantly impacted the therapy of patients with STEMI, with a 19% reduction in PCI procedures leading to increased morbidity and mortality, aspects evidenced also in other studies [34, 40, 43].

3.3 Increased risk of arrhythmias

Arrhythmias were observed precociously in COVID-19 patients worldwide, several centers reporting a large spectrum of electrocardiographic abnormalities [31, 32]. In most cases, sinus tachycardia due to multiple, concomitant causes (hypoperfusion, fever, hypoxia, and anxiety) was observed, but also atrial tachycardia and fibrillation (AF), and less frequently atrioventricular block (AVB) and polymorphic ventricular tachycardia (VT), significantly increasing the morbidity and mortality, and explaining at least in part, the increased number of cardiac arrests noticed in out-of-hospital patients [44, 45]. It was considered that underlying mechanisms are myocardial injury, inflammation, coexisting hypoxia, electrolytic (especially hypokalemia) and acid–base imbalances, and activation of the sympathetic nervous system, which is contributing the medication used to treat this disease such as hydroxychloroquine, azithromycin, and antivirals that prolong the QT interval [46, 47].

Perhaps the most comprehensive study written on this topic is the one of Coromilas et al. who analyzed data collected from over 4000 patients with COVID-19 and arrhythmias, from 4 continents and 12 countries, and concluded that the majority of them (81.8%) developed supraventricular arrhythmias including AF and atrial flutter, 21% of subjects had ventricular arrhythmias, and 22.6% developed bradyarrhythmias [47]. They also observed that arrhythmias were more frequent in patients over 60 years old, male gender prevailed, and frequently systemic hypertension and diabetes mellitus were associated comorbidities [33, 46, 47].

Treatment of arrhythmias should follow the standard guidelines for the management of arrhythmias focusing on the underlying pathophysiological mechanisms, and addressing as much as possible the reversible causes, especially electrolyte abnormalities. In the case of recurrent, uncontrolled ventricular arrhythmias not responding to antiarrhythmic therapy, implantable cardioverter defibrillators may be recommended, and for persistent high-degree AVB transvenous pacemaker insertion [48].

3.4 Thromboembolic events and bleeding risk

As the pandemic unravels, medical literature has provided robust insight into the unique mechanisms of and specific propensity for COVID-19 thrombogenicity, identified as considerably different from other severe infectious and non-infectious diseases. The relationship between SARS-CoV-2 infection and subsequent dysregulation of coagulation homeostasis is reflected in the various rates of occurrence of major venous and arterial thromboembolic/thrombotic events, which, in more extreme cases, have been documented to occur concomitantly. A recent comparative study, which retrospectively evaluated thromboembolic risk in large patient cohorts of COVID-19 and Influenza, found that COVID-19 was independently associated with a higher 90-day risk for venous thrombosis, but not arterial thrombosis, as compared to Influenza, with secondary analysis showing a similar risk for ischemic stroke and myocardial infarction, and a higher risk for deep vein thrombosis (DVT) and pulmonary embolism (PE) in patients with COVID-19 [49].

In spite of early thromboprophylaxis, most frequently, VTE negatively impacts clinical outcomes in COVID-19 hospitalized patients, and the risk seems to be greatest in the intensive care unit (ICU) setting, among the critically ill [50]. Major arterial thrombotic events and VTE have been reported at a higher frequency, in COVID-19 ICU patients, as compared to non-ICU patients, over a 30-day period, despite a thromboprophylaxis rate of 85–90% [51]. Moreover, a recent meta-analysis of 12 studies, in which all patients were under thromboprophylaxis, with either low molecular weight or unfractionated heparin, still showed a 31% pooled prevalence of VTE for ICU admissions [52]. Very recently, an overall incidence of 17.3% for VTE among hospitalized COVID-19 has been reported (~2/3 DVT), with significant discrepancies between pooled incidences of VTE for ICU admissions as compared to general ward patients (27.9% vs. 7.1%, respectively), while including catheter-associated thromboembolism, isolated distal DVT, and isolated pulmonary emboli reached the highest incidence rates. Even so, VTE incidence was higher when assessed within a screening strategy (33.1% vs. 9.8% by clinical diagnosis), meaning that, in clinical practice, it is very likely that many COVID-19 patients with subclinical VTE remain undiagnosed [53]. Moreover, VTE prevalence in COVID-19 patients varies widely depending on the subpopulation evaluated, seemingly correlating well with disease severity and preexisting metabolic and cardiovascular comorbidities, a statement reflected by the variability of occurrence rates reported: <3% in non-ICU patient [51], >30% for ICU cases, with DVT and subsequent PE representing the most common thrombotic complication in the ICU setting [54], while autopsy findings of COVID-19 fatalities suggest it may reach nearly 60% [55].

Interestingly, amounting data suggest that the majority of so-called PE diagnoses occur without a recognizable source of venous embolism and may be better defined as primary in situ pulmonary arterial thrombosis, a direct consequence of the SARS-CoV-2 pulmonary disease, entailing thrombotic occlusion of small–/mid-sized pulmonary arteries, which will result in the infarction of afferent lung parenchyma [56]. This may explain why PE is the most prevalent thrombotic event seen in COVID-19 patients [54] and why screening yielded a higher incidence of VTE than clinical evaluation of asymptomatic patients. In a recent investigation, duplex ultrasound was performed for clinical suspicion of DVT, reporting 41.58% confirmed DVT, 6.93% superficial thrombophlebitis and, surprisingly, 23.76% PE (mostly involving distal pulmonary vessels), yet only 7.92% had PE and concomitant, associated DVT, meaning that 2/3 of PE occurred in the absence of a recognizable DVT, suggesting a causal mechanism of primary thrombosis rather than embolism [56]. Additionally, postmortem analyses of COVID-19 fatalities have frequently documented thrombosis of small- and mid-sized pulmonary arteries, a lesion capable of causing hemorrhagic necrosis, fibrosis, disruption of pulmonary circulation, acute pulmonary hypertension (PH), and ultimately death [55]. Other severe morphopathological modifications of pulmonary tissue architecture have also been frequently reported in COVID-19 autopsy reports, such as severe endothelial injury, with disruption of cell membranes, rampant vascular thrombosis, and significant angiogenesis [25], while other organs also showed microthrombotic lesions on autopsy, but at a lower rate (cardiac thrombi, epicardial coronary artery thrombi and microthrombi in myocardial capillaries, arterioles, and small muscular arteries) [55].

An aforementioned study, analyzing 184 COVID-19 ICU cases, all receiving thromboprophylaxis, demonstrated a 31% cumulative incidence of the defined vascular complication composite outcome (PE, DVT, ischemic stroke, ACS, or systemic arterial embolism). The main independent predictors of thrombotic complications identified were age, with an adjusted hazard ratio (aHR) of 1.05/per year, and coagulopathy [54]. Conversely, regarding VTE, an extensive meta-analysis (44 studies/14,866 hospitalized COVID-19 patients), on the topic acute complications and mortality, reported a much lower prevalence of 15% for VTE, than previously reported. This value may be influenced not only by cohort size but also by other factors such as heterogeneous reporting between the studies evaluated and increased risk of bias, resulting in very low-quality evidence [57].

On the other hand, as seen in the above-mentioned studies, VTE can still occur in noncritically ill COVID-19 patients; therefore, rigorous elaboration of adequate screening and risk stratification protocols for VTE, especially for mild and moderate COVID-19 phenotypes, will be essential, as these patients are much less likely to undergo tromboprophylaxis.

Regarding arterial thromboembolism (ATE), incidence rates among COVID-19 diagnosed patients have consistently been reported as being much lower than for VTE, since the early days of the pandemic (3.7%) to date [54]. Unsettlingly, large-vessel strokes in young and generally healthy people, which became infected with SARS-CoV-2, have been consistently reported [25, 55]. Early retrospective studies, seemingly corroborated these findings, claiming that acute, new-onset, cerebrovascular disease was not uncommon in COVID-19 patients – out 219 consecutive COVID-19 patients, 10 (4.6%) developed acute ischemic stroke and 1 (0.5%) had intracerebral hemorrhage [58] –,and that SARS-CoV-2 infection carried an increased risk of ACS, especially via coronary stent thromboses [59]. Nevertheless, investigations involving a much larger sample size showed that the actual incidence of ATE (thrombotic/embolic) is, in fact, much lower than initially reported in earlier studies [51, 60]. A large cohort retrospective study, evaluating 1114 COVID-19 patients with independently adjudicated thrombotic/embolic events, found stroke and ACS incidence were 0.1% (1/1114) and 1.3% (14/1114), respectively [51]. Most authors agree that thrombotic events occur early in the evolution of COVID-19, and in order to combat the hypercoagulable and prothrombotic state, administration of anticoagulants is recommended to reduce this risk [27].

Of great importance is the fact that, due to several factors such as thrombocytopenia, hyperfibrinolytic state, consumption of coagulation factors, which initiate their action later on, after 1 to 3 weeks, COVID-19 patients may also become prone to bleeding. This must be taken into account, especially in severe COVID-19 cases, where concomitant administration of anticoagulants as thromboprophylaxis is very likely to occur [61]. Additionally, critically ill COVID-19 patients have an even more increased bleeding risk, due to thrombocytopenia/platelet dysfunction or coagulation factor deficiencies, or both [62], which are frequent occurrences in this clinical population. Thus, it has become increasingly difficult to establish an adequate, integrative, anticoagulant prophylaxis strategy for COVID-19.

As opposed to the numerous investigations debating over thromboembolic events, there are much fewer articles focusing on major bleedings and just a few case reports on hematomas in COVID-19. Al-Shamkary et al. reported an overall incidence of 4.8–8% referring to bleeding events, and of 3.5% for major bleedings [62], being mostly associated with advanced age, comorbidities and apparently, more frequent in males.

All in all, thromboembolic events are a frequent morbidity encountered in COVID-19 patients, especially in those with severe forms and comorbidities. For their prophylaxis/treatment anticoagulant therapy is recommended, thus increasing the risk of bleedings. Both thromboembolic events and hemorrhagic complications aggravate the evolution of these patients, representing significant negative prognostic factors and increasing the morbidity and mortality associated with COVID-19.

4. Subacute and long-term cardiovascular sequels following the infection with the SARS-CoV-2 virus

The important contribution of COVID-19 in the pathogenesis of acute cardiovascular involvements is now well established, but because this pandemic is a new disease, long-term data on post-COVID-19 complications were not available [63, 64]. However, more and more studies revealed that the infection with the SARS-CoV-2 virus also causes chronic cardiac complications, even when the viral load is normalized [63, 64], explaining the persistence of symptoms during recovery observed in an increasing number of individuals [65]. In some patients, myocarditis, subacute pericarditis, persisting arrhythmias, pulmonary hypertension, or heart failure have been observed raising serious concerns and indicating that in symptomatic patients, a comprehensive evaluation and a regular long-term follow-up are needed for effective therapeutic regime and to prevent a worse evolution of these cardiovascular complications.

4.1 Pulmonary hypertension

It is well known that pulmonary hypertension (PH) may occur during the acute phase of the SARS-CoV-2 infection as a consequence of extensive lung injury and of altered pulmonary circulation, frequently leading to right heart failure (RHF), shearing common pathophysiological mechanisms with other complications encountered in this illness, and significantly increasing the mortality [66, 67].

In COVID-19 patients, the prevalence of PH varies wildly, depending on the studied population, ranging from 7.69% to 12–13,4% or even 22% in severe COVID-19 cases [67, 68]. While this topic was largely debated in the medical literature, information over its outcome is less available. It has been observed that some patients are predisposed to develop interstitial lung disease (ILD) frequently associated with persisting PH and explaining, at least partially, the persisting symptoms observed in patients with subacute and long COVID-19 [69, 70]. The backgrounds of this disease are complex and multifactorial, including a large variety of pathophysiological types, ranging from arterial PH (group 1), PH of group 3 – due to ILD, to chronic thromboembolism (group 4 PH) or even of group 2 PH (secondary left heart disease) [70, 71]. In their study, Suzuki et al., observed a unique hystopathological finding identified only at the autopsy of COVID-19 patients, namely thickened pulmonary vascular walls, considered an important hallmark of arterial PH [71]. This finding suggests that COVID-19, depending on the severity of the lung injury and the inflammatory responses, could favor the development of PH, and some of these patients may develop in the future signs and symptoms of PH and RHF [71].

The diagnosis of PH is difficult and implies right heart catheterization, which is limited during the pandemic considering the risk of contamination and shortness of personal and resources. In patients infected with SARS-CoV-2, TTE allows an accurate estimation of the systolic pressure in the pulmonary artery, being the most utilized method for the diagnostic and follow-up of these patients. A specific therapy for this type of PH has not been described, and future studies are needed to clarify its management.

4.2 Heart failure

AHF may appear precocious in the evolution of the SARS-CoV-2 infection, in some cases being even the first manifestations. Since COVID-19 and AHF/worsening of CHF shear similar symptoms, distinguishing these two pathologies is challenging, the more so as these two conditions may coexist. Some studies describe an increased prevalence of ACH (23% or even 33%) in patients hospitalized for COVID-19 being associated with an increased risk of mortality [63]. In many cases, it is difficult to establish if AHF is the consequence of a new myocarditis/cardiomyopathy or it represents the exacerbation of previously undiagnosed CHF. Responsible pathophysiological mechanisms of AHF in COVID-19 may include acute myocardial injury due to inflammation (myocarditis), tachyarrhythmia or ischemia, or to acute respiratory failure, acute kidney injury, and hypervolemia [9, 29, 31]. Importantly, RHF may also be present especially in patients with severe pulmonary injury and PE contributing to the increased mortality of these patients [37].

Diagnosis may be difficult, but clinical presentation, history of preexisting cardiovascular comorbidities, evidence of cardiomegaly, and/or bilateral pleural effusion on chest radiography are suggestive. Increased levels of B-type natriuretic peptide (BNP)/N-terminal B-type natriuretic peptide (NT-proBNP) could be an important clue for AHF/worsened CHF, although elevated BNP/NT-proBNP values were also found in COVID-19 patients in the absence of AHF. An important contribution offers TTE demonstrating enlarged cardiac cavities, impaired systolic performance, and other important signs [34, 49, 72].

Therapy of AHF in COVID-19 patients should be performed according to guidelines [63] based on the same recommendation as in subjects without COVID-19, with special attention to early detection and treatment of complications, especially hypoxia, thrombotic/bleeding events, and cardiac arrhythmias. It is important to consider AHF/CHF when administering intravenous fluids avoiding excessive fluid replacement and to be conscious on the cardiac adverse effects of medications used in the treatment of COVID-19 [9, 31, 64].

Referring to patients already diagnosed with CHF, it is well known that they are predisposed to develop more severe forms of COVID-19, being predisposed to a higher mortality. The SARS-CoV-2 infection may also unmask a latent CHF, particularly heart failure with preserved ejection fraction (HFpEF) which is common among elderly overweight, hypertensive patients. In addition, as a consequence of myocardial injury, cardiac fibrosis may occur, explaining the increased frequency of diastolic dysfunction identified on TTE. The risk to develop overt CHF is present both during the acute phase of COVID-19 and during the recovery from the acute illness in survivors [31, 33, 72, 73].

Another aspect is that the COVID-19 pandemic negatively impacted the outcome of patients with CHF who avoided or delayed hospital controls or admissions due to fear of contamination. They presented themselves to the hospital only when their condition was severe, which lead to an increased mortality worldwide [9, 74].

4.3 New onset or aggravation of systemic hypertension

The relationship between the infection with the SARS-CoV-2 virus and systemic hypertension is very complicated and difficult to establish. While it is generally accepted that COVID-19 patients with a history of cardiovascular diseases, especially systemic hypertension, have a worse outcome and increased mortality [29, 75], it is very difficult to establish if there is a new onset or a worsening of a chronic hypertension in the context of this illness, since a previous comprehensive evaluation is not available in the majority of cases. A meta-analysis of Lippi et al. evidenced a nearly 2.5-fold increase of severity and mortality of severe COVID-19 in patients with associated systemic hypertension, especially in those older than 60 years with other comorbidities [75].

Other large meta-analyses focused on the impact of hypertension's severity and its control and the outcomes but failed to document significant connections [76]. It was concluded that hypertension is associated with endothelial dysfunction strongly impacted in COVID-19, and patients with more severe forms have more advanced atherosclerosis and consecutive complications, thus increasing the morbidity and mortality. As the concerns regarding therapy with ACE inhibitors were not found to be justified, treatment should be given according to guidelines to optimize blood pressure values [77].

4.4 Postural orthostatic tachycardiac syndrome

The postural tachycardia syndrome (POTS) is the result of an autonomic dysregulation which determines increased vasoconstriction when standing, resulting in blood pooling within the splanchnic vasculature and limbs, with reduced venous return to the heart. An excessive compensatory tachycardia and increased plasma noradrenaline levels contribute to symptoms, the commonest of which are fatigue, palpitations, light-headedness, headache, and nausea symptoms reported by many of patients with long-COVID (between 15% and 50% according to some studies) [78]. Although orthostatic intolerance is common among patients recovering from a COVID-19 infection, not all have POTS, some of them have only orthostatic hypotension [78].

The exact pathophysiological mechanism of POTS is not fully clarified, and there are several mechanisms involved, including hypovolemia, autonomic denervation, hyperadrenergic stimulation, and autoimmune pathology. It is not well established whether the same recognized pathophysiology of POTS is also present in patients with long COVID further studies being necessary [78].

4.5 Aggravation of preexisting cardiovascular pathologies

From the early stages of the infection with the SARS-CoV-2 virus, it became evident that underlying cardiovascular diseases, obesity, diabetes mellitus, and more advanced age are associated with a higher risk for severe COVID-19 infection [34]. Individuals already suffering from cardiovascular diseases were more likely to be infected with the virus, and the virus infection was likely to determine the deterioration of basic heart disease [79]. Apparently, among COVID-19 patients, there were almost 50% diagnosed with chronic diseases, 40% of them with cardiovascular and cerebrovascular disorders, chronic kidney failure, and chronic obstructive pulmonary disease, having an increased risk of morbidity or even death related to this infection. A large study from the USA reported that the most common comorbidities among patients with COVID-19 were systemic hypertension (56.6%), obesity (41.7%), diabetes (33.8%), coronary artery disease (11.1%), and CHF (6.9%) [33], and a retrospective cohort study in China conducted on patients with cardiovascular comorbidities evidenced a fivefold higher mortality risk (10.5%). Based on these results, hypertension and cardiovascular comorbidities can be considered as risk factors for persons with severe symptoms of the disease.

In COVID-19 cases, it is important to recognize the clinical characteristics of infected persons to identify and effectively treat the associated comorbidities and the newly developed cardiovascular complications as well to reduce patients' morbidity and mortality. Since many antiviral drugs may determine cardiac insufficiency, arrhythmia or other cardiovascular disorders, therefore, during the therapy of this illness, especially with antiviral therapy, the risk of cardiac toxicity needs to be closely monitored [79].

Another aspect is that of the long-term outcome of patients who suffered from a SARS-CoV-2 infection. In a recent and comprehensive study realized on over 150000 individuals recovering from COVID-19 [80], Xie et al. highlighted that beyond the first month after infection, people with COVID-19 experienced at 12 months an increased morbidity risks and burdens of cardiovascular diseases, including cerebrovascular disorders, dysrhythmias, inflammatory heart disease, ischemic heart disease, heart failure, thromboembolic disease, and other cardiac disorders [80]. These risks were obvious regardless of age, race, gender, and associated cardiovascular risk factors, including obesity, hypertension, diabetes, chronic kidney disease, and hyperlipidemia, being evident even in individuals without history of cardiovascular pathology before the SARS-CoV-2 virus infection, raising concerns that these risks might be present even in people at low risk of cardiovascular disease [80]. These risks and associated burdens increased parallel to the severity of the acute phase of COVID-19: from non-hospitalized individuals – who were the majority – to hospitalized patients, especially to those admitted to the intensive care units [80].

4.6 Cardiovascular effects of medication used to treat COVID-19

It has been observed that many of the medications used for the treatment of COVID-19 strongly interfere with other medications used in the therapy of cardiovascular diseases, such as anticoagulants, antiplatelets, statins, antihypertensives, and especially antiarrhythmics favoring the occurrence of arrhythmias [31]. Some antibiotics (azithromycin), corticosteroids, antimalarials (chloroquine, hydroxychloroquine), newly developed therapies, still under study such as antivirals (remdesivir, ribavirin, lopinavir/ritonavir, and favipiravir), and biologics (tocilizumab) determine cardiotoxicity, interact with electrolyte metabolism, and many of them, especially Lopinavir/ritonavir, may cause QT and PR prolongation favoring the occurrence of arrhythmias or conduction disturbances, mainly in patients already treated with drugs prolonging the QT interval. Data over the mechanism of action and potential effects of main medication used in the treatment of COVID-19 is presented in **Table 1** [31].

4.7 Cardiovascular effects related to vaccination

After the introduction of mRNA COVID-19 vaccines a higher incidence of myocarditis in vaccine recipients. A study performed on the data basis from an Israeli national database concluded that the incidence of myocarditis after two doses of the BNT162b2 mRNA vaccine was reduced (risk ratio = 3.24), significantly lower than after COVID-19 (risk ratio = 18.28), but higher than in unvaccinated individuals. The risk of myocarditis was higher after the second dose of vaccine and in young male recipients [81].

Similar results were also reported by other researcher, with an elevated risk of myocarditis, pericarditis, and myopericarditis observed particularly among young males with 39–47 expected cases of per million second mRNA COVID-19 vaccine

Medication	Mechanism of action	Cardiovascular effects and drug interactions
Azithromycin	Interacts with the synthesis of proteins and binds to 50s ribosome	• Interferes with statins, anticoagulants, and antiarrhythmics, prolonging QT interval and favoring arrhythmias (torsades de pointes).
Chloroquine and Hydroxychloroquine	Alterations in the pH of endosomal/organelle	• May induce direct myocardial toxicity worsening myocarditis and cardiomyopathy. • Alter intracardiac conduction resulting in bundle branch block, AV block. • Interact with antiarrhythmics favoring ventricular arrhythmias, torsades de pointes.
Methylprednisolone	Anti-inflammatory	• Determines fluid retention, hypertension, and dyselectrolytemia. • Interacts with anticoagulants.
Remdesivir	Inhibitor of RNA polymerases	• May cause hypotension and arrhythmias.
Ribavirin	Inhibits RNA and DNA virus replication	• Interacts with anticoagulants. • May cause severe hemolytic anemia.
Lopinavir/Ritonavir	Lopinavir inhibits protease and Ritonavir inhibits CYP3A metabolism	• Interacts with anticoagulants, antiplatelets, statins, and antiarrhythmics. • May determine prolonged QT interval, AV blocks, and torsades de pointes.
Favipiravir	Inhibits RNA-dependent RNA polymerases	• Interacts with anticoagulants, statins, and antiarrhythmics.
Interferon	Immune system activation	• May determine direct myocardial toxicity. • Worsens cardiomyopathy; alters intracardiac conduction. • Causes hypotension or cardiac ischemia.
Tocilizumab	Inhibits IL-6	• May interfere with some medication metabolism such as statins. • May determine hypertension.

Table 1.
Interactions of medications used in the treatment of COVID-19.

doses administered [82]. They reported an increased risk of myocarditis after the first dose of ChAdOx1 and BNT162b2 vaccines and the first and second doses of the mRNA-1273 vaccine [82].

5. Conclusions

The impairment of the cardiovascular system in COVID-19 comprises a wide spectrum of dysfunctions, ranging from mild to severe, or even life-threatening forms, often having an acute onset, sometimes continuing during recovery or even resulting in chronic pathologies. Individuals are affected regardless of age, race, gender, and associated cardiovascular risk factors, but those with a history of cardiovascular pathology prior to the SARS-CoV-2 virus infection have a worse outcome. Therefore, a comprehensive cardiologic evaluation, including TTE, is justified to assess the involvement of the cardiovascular system, for initiating a proper therapy as soon as possible and to schedule a follow-up program particularly in patients at high risk.

Author details

Cristina Tudoran*, Mariana Tudoran, Voichita Elena Lazureanu,
Adelina Raluca Marinescu, Dorin Novacescu and Talida Georgiana Cut
University of Medicine and Pharmacy "Victor Babeş", Timişoara, Romania

*Address all correspondence to: tudoran.mariana@umft.ro

References

[1] WHO Director-General's Opening Remarks at the Media Briefing on COVID-19-11 March 2020. [cited April 27, 2021]. Available from: https://www.who.int/director-general/speeches/detail/who-director-general-s-opening-remarks-at-the-media-briefing-on-covid-19---11-march-2020

[2] COVID Live—Coronavirus Statistics—Worldometer. [cited February 11, 2022]. Available from: https://www.worldometers.info/coronavirus/

[3] Dumache R, Daescu E, Ciocan V, Mureşan C, Talida C, Gavrilita D, et al. Molecular testing of SARS-CoV-2 infection from blood samples in disseminated intravascular coagulation (DIC) and elevated D-dimer levels. Clinical Laboratory. 2021;**67**(1):187-192

[4] Harrison AG, Lin T, Wang P. Mechanisms of SARS-CoV-2 Transmission and Pathogenesis. Trends in Immunology. 2020;**41**(12):1100-1115

[5] Ziegler CGK, Allon SJ, Nyquist SK, Mbano IM, Miao VN, Tzouanas CN, et al. SARS-CoV-2 Receptor ACE2 is an interferon-stimulated gene in human airway epithelial cells and is detected in specific cell subsets across tissues. Cell. 2020;**181**(5):1016-1035

[6] Zhao Y, Zhao Z, Wang Y, Zhou Y, Ma Y, Zuo W. Single-cell RNA expression profiling of ACE2, the receptor of SARS-CoV-2. American Journal of Respiratory and Critical Care Medicine. 2020;**202**(5):756-759

[7] Varga Z, Flammer AJ, Steiger P, Haberecker M, Andermatt R, Zinkernagel AS, et al. Endothelial cell infection and endotheliitis in COVID-19. Lancet. 2020;**395**(10234):1417-1418

[8] Leentjens J, van Haaps TF, Wessels PF, Schutgens REG, Middeldorp S. COVID-19-associated coagulopathy and antithrombotic agents—lessons after 1 year. The Lancet Haematology. 2021;**8**(7):e524-e533

[9] Italia L, Tomasoni D, Bisegna S, Pancaldi E, Stretti L, Adamo M, et al. COVID-19 and Heart Failure: From Epidemiology During the Pandemic to Myocardial Injury, Myocarditis, and Heart Failure Sequelae. Frontiers in Cardiovascular Medicine. 2021;**8**:1-14

[10] Tomasoni D, Italia L, Adamo M, Inciardi RM, Lombardi CM, Solomon SD, et al. COVID-19 and heart failure: From infection to inflammation and angiotensin II stimulation. Searching for evidence from a new disease. European Journal of Heart Failure. 2020;**22**(6):957-966

[11] Zheng Y-Y, Ma Y-T, Zhang J-Y, Xie X. COVID-19 and the cardiovascular system. Nature Reviews: Cardiology. 2020;**17**(5):259-260

[12] Lindner D, Fitzek A, Bräuninger H, Aleshcheva G, Edler C, Meissner K, et al. Association of cardiac infection with SARS-CoV-2 in confirmed COVID-19 autopsy cases. JAMA Cardiology. 2020;**5**(11):1-5

[13] Patel VB, Zhong J-C, Grant MB, Oudit GY. Role of the ACE2/Angiotensin 1-7 axis of the renin-angiotensin system in heart failure. Circulation Research. 2016;**118**(8):1313-1326

[14] Madjid M, Safavi-Naeini P, Solomon SD, Vardeny O. Potential effects of coronaviruses on the cardiovascular system: A review. JAMA Cardiology. 2020;**5**(7):831-840

[15] Ragab D, Salah Eldin H, Taeimah M, Khattab R, Salem R. The COVID-19 cytokine storm; what we know so far. Frontiers in Immunology. 2020;**11**:1446

[16] Tay MZ, Poh CM, Rénia L, MacAry PA, Ng LFP. The trinity of COVID-19: Immunity, inflammation and intervention. Nature Reviews. Immunology. 2020;**20**(6):363-374

[17] Guo Y-R, Cao Q-D, Hong Z-S, Tan Y-Y, Chen S-D, Jin H-J, et al. The origin, transmission and clinical therapies on coronavirus disease 2019 (COVID-19) outbreak – An update on the status. Military Medical Research. 2020;**7**(1):11

[18] Huang C, Wang Y, Li X, Ren L, Zhao J, Hu Y, et al. Clinical features of patients infected with 2019 novel coronavirus in Wuhan, China. The Lancet. 2020;**395**(10223):497-506

[19] Zhou Y, Fu B, Zheng X, Wang D, Zhao C, Qi Y, et al. Pathogenic T cells and inflammatory monocytes incite inflammatory storm in severe COVID-19 patients. National Science Review. 2020;**7**(6):998-1002

[20] Yang X, Yu Y, Xu J, Shu H, Xia J, Liu H, et al. Clinical course and outcomes of critically ill patients with SARS-CoV-2 pneumonia in Wuhan, China: A single-centered, retrospective, observational study. The Lancet Respiratory Medicine. 2020;**8**(5):475-481

[21] Shi S, Qin M, Shen B, Cai Y, Liu T, Yang F, et al. Association of cardiac injury with mortality in hospitalized patients with COVID-19 in Wuhan, China. JAMA Cardiology. 2020;**5**(7):802-810

[22] Arévalos V, Ortega-Paz L, Rodríguez-Arias JJ, Calvo M, Castrillo L, Salazar A, et al. Myocardial injury in COVID-19 patients: Association with inflammation, coagulopathy and in-hospital prognosis. Journal of Clinical Medicine. 2021;**10**(10):2096

[23] Joulin O, Petillot P, Labalette M, Lancel S, Neviere R. Cytokine profile of human septic shock serum inducing cardiomyocyte contractile dysfunction. Physiological Research. 2007;**56**(3):291-297

[24] Unudurthi SD, Luthra P, Bose RJC, McCarthy JR, Kontaridis MI. Cardiac inflammation in COVID-19: Lessons from heart failure. Life Sciences. 2020;**260**:118482

[25] Ackermann M, Verleden SE, Kuehnel M, Haverich A, Welte T, Laenger F, et al. Pulmonary vascular endothelialitis, thrombosis, and angiogenesis in Covid-19. The New England Journal of Medicine. 2020;**383**(2):120-128

[26] Fajnzylber J, Regan J, Coxen K, Corry H, Wong C, Rosenthal A, et al. SARS-CoV-2 viral load is associated with increased disease severity and mortality. Nature Communications. 2020;**11**(1):5493

[27] Bikdeli B, Madhavan MV, Jimenez D, Chuich T, Dreyfus I, Driggin E, et al. COVID-19 and thrombotic or thromboembolic disease: Implications for prevention, antithrombotic therapy, and follow-up: JACC State-of-the-Art Review. Journal of the American College of Cardiology. 2020;**75**(23):2950-2973

[28] Singhania N, Bansal S, Nimmatoori DP, Ejaz AA, McCullough PA, Singhania G. Current overview on hypercoagulability in COVID-19. American Journal of Cardiovascular Drugs. 2020;**20**(5):393-403

[29] Farshidfar F, Koleini N, Ardehali H. Cardiovascular

complications of COVID-19. JCI Insight. 2021;**6**(13):1-15

[30] Lewek J, Jatczak-Pawlik I, Maciejewski M, Jankowski P, Banach M. COVID-19 and cardiovascular complications – The preliminary results of the LATE-COVID study. Archives of Medical Science. 2021;**17**(3):818-822

[31] Long B, Brady WJ, Koyfman A, Gottlieb M. Cardiovascular complications in COVID-19. The American Journal of Emergency Medicine. 2020;**38**(7):1504-1507

[32] Ranard LS, Fried JA, Abdalla M, Anstey DE, Givens RC, Kumaraiah D, et al. Approach to acute cardiovascular complications in COVID-19 infection. Circulation. 2020;**13**(7):e007220

[33] Guzik TJ, Mohiddin SA, Dimarco A, Patel V, Savvatis K, Marelli-Berg FM, et al. COVID-19 and the cardiovascular system: Implications for risk assessment, diagnosis, and treatment options. Cardiovascular Research. 2020;**116**(10):1666-1687

[34] The Task Force for the management of COVID-19 of the European Society of Cardiology, Baigent C, Windecker S, Andreini D, Arbelo E, Barbato E, et al. ESC guidance for the diagnosis and management of cardiovascular disease during the COVID-19 pandemic: Part 2—care pathways, treatment, and follow-up. European Heart Journal. 2021;**43**(11):1033-1058

[35] Tung-Chen Y. Acute pericarditis due to COVID-19 infection: An underdiagnosed disease? Medicina Clínica (Barcelona). 2020;**155**(1): 44-45

[36] Diaz-Arocutipa C, Saucedo-Chinchay J, Imazio M. Pericarditis in patients with COVID-19: A systematic review. Journal of Cardiovascular Medicine. 2021;**22**(9):693-700

[37] Tudoran C, Tudoran M, Pop GN, Giurgi-Oncu C, Cut TG, Lazureanu VE, et al. Associations between the Severity of the Post-Acute COVID-19 Syndrome and Echocardiographic Abnormalities in Previously Healthy Outpatients Following Infection with SARS-CoV-2. Biology. 2021;**10**(6):469

[38] Ashraf S, Ilyas S, Alraies MC. Acute coronary syndrome in the time of the COVID-19 pandemic. European Heart Journal. 2020;**41**(22):2089-2091

[39] Mafham MM, Spata E, Goldacre R, Gair D, Curnow P, Bray M, et al. COVID-19 pandemic and admission rates for and management of acute coronary syndromes in England. The Lancet. 2020;**396**(10248):381-389

[40] Zaleski AL, Taylor BA, McKay RG, Thompson PD. Declines in acute cardiovascular emergencies during the COVID-19 pandemic. The American Journal of Cardiology. 2020;**129**:124-125

[41] Mahmud E, Dauerman HL, Welt FGP, Messenger JC, Rao SV, Grines C, et al. Management of acute myocardial infarction during the COVID -19 pandemic: A Consensus Statement from the Society for Cardiovascular Angiography and Interventions (SCAI), the American College of Cardiology (ACC), and the American College of Emergency Physicians (ACEP). Catheterization and Cardiovascular Interventions. 2020;**96**(2):336-345

[42] Fileti L, Vecchio S, Moretti C, Reggi A, Aquilina M, Balducelli M, et al. Impact of the COVID-19 pandemic on coronary invasive procedures at two Italian high-volume referral centers. Journal of Cardiovascular Medicine. 2020;**21**(11):869-873

[43] De Luca G, Verdoia M, Cercek M, Jensen LO, Vavlukis M, Calmac L, et al. Impact of COVID-19 pandemic on mechanical reperfusion for patients with STEMI. Journal of the American College of Cardiology. 2020;**76**(20):2321-2330

[44] Kochav SM, Coromilas E, Nalbandian A, Ranard LS, Gupta A, Chung MK, et al. Cardiac arrhythmias in COVID-19 infection. Circulation: Arrhythmia and Electrophysiology. 2020;**13**(6):e008719

[45] Kochi AN, Tagliari AP, Forleo GB, Fassini GM, Tondo C. Cardiac and arrhythmic complications in patients with COVID-19. Journal of Cardiovascular Electrophysiology. 2020;**31**(5):1003-1008

[46] Patel NH, Rutland J, Tecson KM. Arrhythmias and intraventricular conduction disturbances in patients hospitalized with coronavirus disease 2019. The American Journal of Cardiology. 2022;**162**:111-115

[47] Coromilas EJ, Kochav S, Goldenthal I, Biviano A, Garan H, Goldbarg S, et al. Worldwide survey of COVID-19–associated arrhythmias. Circulation: Arrhythmia and Electrophysiology. 2021; **14**(3):e009458

[48] Lakkireddy DR, Chung MK, Gopinathannair R, Patton KK, Gluckman TJ, Turagam M, et al. Guidance for cardiac electrophysiology during the COVID-19 pandemic from the Heart Rhythm Society COVID-19 Task Force; Electrophysiology Section of the American College of Cardiology; and the Electrocardiography and Arrhythmias Committee of the Council on Clinical Cardiology. American Heart Association. Heart Rhythm. 2020;**17**(9):e233-e241

[49] Ward A, Sarraju A, Lee D, Bhasin K, Gad S, Beetel R, et al. COVID-19 is associated with higher risk of venous thrombosis, but not arterial thrombosis, compared with influenza: Insights from a large US Cohort. PLoS One. 2022;**17**(1):e0261786

[50] Fontana P, Casini A, Robert-Ebadi H, Glauser F, Righini M, Blondon M. Venous thromboembolism in COVID-19: Systematic review of reported risks and current guidelines. Swiss Medical Weekly. 2020;**150**:w20301

[51] Piazza G, Campia U, Hurwitz S, Snyder JE, Rizzo SM, Pfeferman MB, et al. Registry of arterial and venous thromboembolic complications in patients with COVID-19. Journal of the American College of Cardiology. 2020;**76**(18):2060-2072

[52] Hasan SS, Radford S, Kow CS, Zaidi STR. Venous thromboembolism in critically ill COVID-19 patients receiving prophylactic or therapeutic anticoagulation: A systematic review and meta-analysis. Journal of Thrombosis and Thrombolysis. 2020;**50**(4):814-821

[53] Jiménez D, García-Sanchez A, Rali P, Muriel A, Bikdeli B, Ruiz-Artacho P, et al. Incidence of VTE and bleeding among hospitalized patients with coronavirus disease 2019. Chest. 2021;**159**(3):1182-1196

[54] Klok FA, Kruip MJHA, van der Meer NJM, Arbous MS, Gommers DAMPJ, Kant KM, et al. Incidence of thrombotic complications in critically ill ICU patients with COVID-19. Thrombosis Research. 2020;**191**:145-147

[55] Wichmann D, Sperhake J-P, Lütgehetmann M, Steurer S, Edler C, Heinemann A, et al. Autopsy findings and venous thromboembolism in patients with COVID-19. Annals of Internal Medicine. 2020;**6**:M20

[56] Marone EM, Bonalumi G, Curci R, Arzini A, Chierico S, Marazzi G, et al. Characteristics of venous thromboembolism in COVID-19 patients: A multicenter experience from Northern Italy. Annals of Vascular Surgery. 2020;**68**:83-87

[57] Potere N, Valeriani E, Candeloro M, Tana M, Porreca E, Abbate A, et al. Acute complications and mortality in hospitalized patients with coronavirus disease 2019: A systematic review and meta-analysis. Critical Care. 2020;**24**:389

[58] Li Y, Li M, Wang M, Zhou Y, Chang J, Xian Y, et al. Acute cerebrovascular disease following COVID-19: A single center, retrospective, observational study. Stroke Vascular Neurology. 2020;**5**(3):279-284

[59] Prieto-Lobato A, Ramos-Martínez R, Vallejo-Calcerrada N, Corbí-Pascual M, Córdoba-Soriano JG. A case series of stent thrombosis during the COVID-19 pandemic. JACC Case Reports. 2020;**2**(9):1291-1296

[60] Bilaloglu S, Aphinyanaphongs Y, Jones S, Iturrate E, Hochman J, Berger JS. Thrombosis in hospitalized patients with COVID-19 in a New York City Health System. Journal of the American Medical Association. 2020;**324**(8):799-801

[61] Becker RC. COVID-19 update: Covid-19-associated coagulopathy. Journal of Thrombosis and Thrombolysis. 2020;**50**(1):54-67

[62] Al-Samkari H, Karp Leaf RS, Dzik WH, Carlson JCT, Fogerty AE, Waheed A, et al. COVID-19 and coagulation: Bleeding and thrombotic manifestations of SARS-CoV-2 infection. Blood. 2020;**136**(4):489-500

[63] Szekely Y, Lichter Y, Taieb P, Banai A, Hochstadt A, Merdler I, et al. Spectrum of cardiac manifestations in COVID-19: A Systematic Echocardiographic Study. Circulation. 2020;**142**(4):342-353

[64] MVB| NW| CN|. Research Reveals Heart Complications in COVID-19 Patients. CIDRAP; 2020 [cited October 31, 2020]. Available from: https://www.cidrap.umn.edu/news-perspective/2020/07/research-reveals-heart-complications-covid-19-patients

[65] Iqubal A, Iqubal MK, Hoda F, Najmi AK, Haque SE. COVID-19 and cardiovascular complications: An update from the underlying mechanism to consequences and possible clinical intervention. Expert Review of Anti Infective Therapy. **19**(9):1083-1092

[66] Mishra A, Lal A, Sahu KK, George AA, Martin K, Sargent J. An update on pulmonary hypertension in coronavirus disease-19 (COVID-19): Pulmonary hypertension and COVID -19. Acta Bio-Medica. 2020;**91**(4):e2020155

[67] Khan AW, Ullah I, Khan KS, Tahir MJ, Masyeni S, Harapan H. Pulmonary arterial hypertension post COVID-19: A sequala of SARS-CoV-2 infection? Respiratory Medicine Case Reports. 2021;**33**:101429

[68] Pagnesi M, Baldetti L, Beneduce A, Calvo F, Gramegna M, Pazzanese V, et al. Pulmonary hypertension and right ventricular involvement in hospitalised patients with COVID-19. Heart. 2020;**106**(17):1324-1331

[69] Aronson KI, Podolanczuk AJ. Lungs after COVID-19: Evolving knowledge of post–COVID-19 interstitial lung disease. Annals ATS. 2021;**18**(5):773-774

[70] Potus F, Mai V, Lebret M, Malenfant S, Breton-Gagnon E, Lajoie AC, et al. Novel insights on the pulmonary vascular consequences

of COVID-19. American Journal of Physiology. Lung Cellular and Molecular Physiology. 2020;**319**(2):L277-L288

[71] Suzuki YJ, Nikolaienko SI, Shults NV, Gychka SG. COVID-19 patients may become predisposed to pulmonary arterial hypertension. Medical Hypotheses. 2021;**147**:110483

[72] Tudoran M, Tudoran C, Lazureanu VE, Marinescu AR, Pop GN, Pescariu AS, et al. Alterations of left ventricular function persisting during post-acute COVID-19 in subjects without previously diagnosed cardiovascular pathology. Journal of Personalized Medicine. 2021;**11**:225-232

[73] Baycan OF, Barman HA, Atici A, Tatlisu A, Bolen F, Ergen P, et al. Evaluation of biventricular function in patients with COVID-19 using speckle tracking echocardiography. International Journal of Cardiovascular Imaging. 2020;**37**(1):135-144

[74] Rey JR, Caro-Codón J, Rosillo SO, Iniesta ÁM, Castrejón-Castrejón S, Marco-Clement I, et al. Heart failure in COVID-19 patients: Prevalence, incidence and prognostic implications. European Journal of Heart Failure. 2020;**22**(12):2205-2215

[75] Lippi G, Wong J, Henry BM. Hypertension in patients with coronavirus disease 2019 (COVID-19): A pooled analysis. Polish Archives of Internal Medicine. 2020;**130**(4):304-309

[76] Sheppard JP, Nicholson BD, Lee J, McGagh D, Sherlock J, Koshiaris C, et al. Association between blood pressure control and coronavirus disease 2019 outcomes in 45 418 symptomatic patients with hypertension: An Observational Cohort Study. Hypertension. 2021;**77**(3): 846-855

[77] World Health Organization. Guideline for the Pharmacological Treatment of Hypertension in Adults. Geneva: World Health Organization; 2021 [cited February 8, 2022]. Available from: https://apps.who.int/iris/handle/10665/344424

[78] Kavi L. Postural tachycardia syndrome and long COVID: An update. The British Journal of General Practice. 2022;**72**(714):8-9

[79] Naeini MB, Sahebi M, Nikbakht F, Jamshidi Z, Ahmadimanesh M, Hashemi M, et al. A meta-meta-analysis: Evaluation of meta-analyses published in the effectiveness of cardiovascular comorbidities on the severity of COVID-19. Obesity Medicine. 2021;**22**:100323

[80] Xie Y, Xu E, Bowe B, Al-Aly Z. Long-term cardiovascular outcomes of COVID-19. Nature Medicine. 2022

[81] Mevorach D, Anis E, Cedar N, Bromberg M, Haas EJ, Nadir E, et al. Myocarditis after BNT162b2 mRNA vaccine against Covid-19 in Israel. The New England Journal of Medicine. 2021;**385**(23):2140-2149

[82] Patone M, Mei XW, Handunnetthi L, Dixon S, Zaccardi F, Shankar-Hari M, et al. Risks of myocarditis, pericarditis, and cardiac arrhythmias associated with COVID-19 vaccination or SARS-CoV-2 infection. Nature Medicine. 2021

Chapter 8

Ageing and HIV-Risk in Non-Gravid Female Humans

Kelvin Leshabari, Godfrey Chale and Rashid Salim

Abstract

Objective: To estimate the association between ageing process markers (e.g. clinical conditions necessitating total abdominal hysterectomy) and immune functions (i.e. HIV-risk) among adult non-gravid female humans. **Materials & Methods:** We did a secondary data analysis, from a prospective, observational, hospital-based study conducted in Dar es Salaam, Tanzania. The primary study population included all women planned for Total Abdominal Hysterectomy (TAH). Target population was all women who underwent TAH. Data were analysed using a generalized linear model via SAS statistical software version 9.4. **Results:** We analysed 40981 women-hours of follow-up. None of the participant seroconverted against HIV during follow-up period, making an HIV-incidence of 0/40981 women-hours. All participants were black Africans (median age 42 (IQR: 37–47) years). We found a statistically significant drop (aOR: 0.687) in HIV-risk after age of 45 years. Serial correlation between age and HIV-serostatus was found ($\gamma = -0.514$, $P = 0.000$). Association between HIV and marital stata was barely significant ($\chi^2 = 8.0176$, df = 3). **Conclusion:** There was a statistically significant reduced HIV-risk after the age of 45 years among hysterectomised women up and above the known behavioural/clinical risks. Participants who reported married had the highest HIV-seropositivity rate. **Recommendations:** These findings reflect antagonistic pleiotropy theory of ageing. Analyses on potential biological mechanism(s) against HIV in peri/post-menopausal women is/are warranted.

Keywords: ageing, antagonistic pleiotropy, endocrinology, hysterectomy, prospective, Dar es Salaam

1. Introduction

There is no doubt that human reproductive endocrine hormones display a handful of mysterious patterns in their ageing process. The patterns are debatable even among endocrinologists and physiologists alike. We did a secondary analysis of findings, to quantify part of the mysterious association, *of ageing process (surgical removal of endocrine uteri) and immune functions (HIV-risk) in non-gravid adult female humans*. Categorically, we asked ourselves whether there is any significant relationship between female reproductive endocrinology and HIV-pathobiology given the ageing process. We believe there is an unaccounted function(s) of reproductive hormones and HIV-pathogenesis in humans. Besides, the unknown function(s) seem(s) to function in a manner that is at present mysterious given the current scientific knowledge base. We also considered the mystery to be descriptive to a number of other ageing related pathologies. The systemic reproductive endocrine mysteries reflect both structure and functions. At functional level, there exist frequent speculations, about mysterious benefits of endogenous progesterone (and even oestradiol?), against bacterial and viral invasions, along the reproductive tissues and cells. Otherwise, it is common knowledge in mammalian female embryology and anatomy, that during embryo-fetal development, premordial germ cells migrate, from the yolk sac to the gonadal ridge, and statistically populate the gonads. The movement is characterised by changes of the premordial germ cells into oogonia, in an unknown mechanism to science, even to the present day. Oogonia rearrange themselves into germ cell nests. These germ cell nests undergo a series of mitotic divisions. Oogonia enters 1st meiotic division as primary oocytes with arrest at diplotene stage until puberty. What exactly triggers those structural processes is still a mystery among scholars to date. The magic behind female mammalian reproductive endocrinology is not confined to structure.

There is palpable evidence to suggest that mammalian endocrine reproductive system is associated with a number of immune functions, some potentially beneficial against viral illnesses [1–4]. However, the concept of endocrine reproductive (dys)-functions against HIV infection in humans is only poorly understood [5]. For instance, Polis and colleagues have reported up to a 40% increased risk of HIV acquisition [6], associated with usage of progestin-based injectable contraceptives in adult females, specifically Depot Medroxy Progesterone Acetate (DMPA) [6]. However, much as the effects of potential confounding could not be completely ruled out in their study findings, it was still an interesting observation to our research group. Specifically, it followed logic, to check whether the same observation, was applicable to endogenous produced progesterone, in non-gravid state. Besides, most physiological functions of endocrine activities, and their effects on immune system, have been studied in adult males. Thus, the gap about the situation in adult females is widening, especially in the era of viral pandemics like SARS COV-2 and HIV/AIDS. It was on this basis, we hypothesised that *the female uterus, and its associated secretory functions, to be an important milieu, for enhancing HIV acquisition in humans*.

A number of actions displayed by female human reproductive system are associated with ageing process. For instance, it is still debatable among endocrinologists, on *how does the menstrual cycle coordinate itself, and cease to function after calendar time*, using hypothalamic-pituitary-gonadal axis. Besides, the uterine endometrium coordinates a handful of both reproductive and immunologic functions. Of importance to this chapter, uterine macrophages and epithelial cells have been shown to be key allies in mobilisation of innate defenses over calendar age [7, 8]. However, the exact cause behind the observation remains a matter of intellectual guess work among scientists to date. We hypothesized the observation to be related to probable endogenous progesterone and/or oestradiol effects.

Information on the relationship between gestation process in humans and HIV-infection is evident in published literature [9–14], and new information still accumulates rapidly [15–18]. Previous studies pinpointed potential biological mechanisms between endocrinology (i.e. endogenous oestradiol and progesterone effects) and immunobiology of HIV [4, 5]. However, most of this accumulated information tends to be biased due to samples used; characterised to be in gestational period, and therefore in an *altered physiologic state*. Little (if any) is known, about the contribution of endocrine functions, towards HIV-risk and HIV-disease process in normal physiological states. To avoid biases associated with '*altered physiological processes*' prominent in gestational era, usage of non-gravid female humans, preferably after reproductive era, becomes justified.

There exists evidence about sex differences in immune responses among adult humans [1], but it is still not clear, the extent contributed by sex hormones, especially among adult female humans, in non-gravid state. We believe that, *there exists differential deleterious effects of female endogenous sex hormones, on HIV risks in non-gravid adult female human population*. However, to the best of our knowledge, the findings of this concept has not been evident in published literature to date.

Hysterectomy can simply be defined as *a surgical removal of the female uterus*. It can also include removal of adjacent structures (e.g. cervix) as evident in *total abdominal hysterectomy* and/or fallopian tubes and ovaries (*hysterectomy with (uni)-bilateral salpingo-oophorectomy*). Hysterectomy is the commonest gynaecologic surgery reported globally [19, 20]. We considered it as a natural surrogate equivalent of non-gravid state in our study cohort. Specifically, it offers a convenient platform, for analysing clinical and biological parameters associated with surgery, exclusively in non-gravid state. Effects of HIV on surgical indications and outcomes among women have been almost exclusively confined to Caesarean section. Caesarean section is an obstetric surgical procedure. Normal physiology in women, and their alterations in early stages of pathologic processes, can be best studied in non-gravid state. Thus, the quest for the interplay between female endocrine reproductive hormones (e.g. oestradiol and progesterone) and HIV pathobiology in non-gravid state remains unknown to the world of science. It was on this basis, we considered hysterectomised women as a natural reservoir to test our beliefs using a clinical research design and adopting specified statistical techniques in our hypothesis testing.

2. Methods

We did a secondary data analysis from a prospective, facility-based follow-up study, at all public regional referral hospitals in Dar-es- Salaam, Tanzania. Specifically, the study took place at Amana, Mwananyamala and Temeke regional referral hospitals. It was conceived as a clinical research study that assessed indications and outcomes of TAH in Dar es Salaam city, Tanzania. Dar-es-Salaam is a cosmopolitan city situated on the East-African coast. It is the business capital of Tanzania. The same city is projected to be 10th largest city on earth in population size come 2050. Geo-strategically, Dar-es-Salaam is a port city, and home to dozens of African demographic subsets, ranging from mainly the Bantu population group to African-Arabic mixed race population.

Data in the primary study was collected using a pre-designed clinical sheet that contained social, demographic, biological and clinical parameters on pre- and peri-480-hours post-hysterectomy. Specifically, HIV screening was accomplished using a serial algorithm involving SD Bioline HIV kit (SD Bioline HIV 1/2 3.0, Standard Diagnostics, Korea) to all participants. Those who were reactive on SD Bioline HIV test, confirmatory diagnosis was made using Unigold HIV kit (UniGold™HIV, Trinity Biotech Manufacturing Ltd, Bray-Ireland). Each participant was screened twice, first at the time of recruitment into the study, and again either before discharge from the ward post-operatively or anytime within 480-hours post-hysterectomy. Data collection started immediately upon a verbal informed consent for inclusion into the primary study. Sample size was obtained using the prospective cohort formula from Kasiulevicius and others publication in the journal Gerontology back in 2006 [21];

$$\text{Sample size} = \frac{\left[\frac{Z_{\alpha}\sqrt{\left(1+\frac{1}{m}\right)p^*(1-p^*)} + Z_{\beta}\sqrt{p1}}{(1-p1)/m + p2(1-p2)} \right]^2}{(p_1 - p_2)^2}$$

Z_{α} = Standard normal variate for level of significance.
m = Number of control subject per experimental subject.
Z_{β} = Standard normal variate for power or type 2 error as explained in earlier section.
$p1$ = Probability of events in control group.
$p2$ = Probability of events in experimental group p

$$P^* = \frac{p2 + mp1}{m+1}$$

For values of Z = 1.96, α = 0.05, β = 0.8, m = 1.

Study population in the primary study included all women with a surrogate marker for *ageing process* (clinical indications necessitating total abdominal hysterectomy). Target population referred to all women who underwent *total abdominal hysterectomy* at any of Dar es Salaam Public Regional Referral Hospitals. Thus, for a participant to be eligible for recruitment into the study, she had to be planned for *total abdominal hysterectomy* and/or emergency total abdominal hysterectomy due to a decision made on the operation table (in-theatre major adverse events) out of another planned surgery at any of those facilities during the study time. All women who underwent sub-total hysterectomies were thus excluded. The decision to do so originated from the assumption that, *for a woman to be planned for total abdominal hysterectomy, the clinical decision rule must incorporate a pathology associated with what we characterized as an ageing process*. Participants were recruited upon official notification for total abdominal hysterectomy at clinics (outpatients) or wards (inpatients) after clinical indications. Participants were followed-up to at most 480-hours post-operatively, or upon discharge from the ward post-operatively, whichever came first. Follow-up data included post-operative HIV serostata.

Data analysis was done using SAS software version 9.4 (SAS Institute, Cary-NC, USA). A minimum number of 106 women had at least 80% power of detecting a statistically significant difference at apriori 5% α-level. Continuous variables were summarised using median (with inter-quartile range). Categorical variables were summarized as proportion (with %). A generalised linear model was used to analyse data after appropriate validation of model assumptions. We considered at least 110 women as a rough estimate of effective sample size in cases of any potential refusal to participate/missing data. However, efforts were made to ensure minimal refusals to participate/missing information per participant via adoption of all surgical and nursing team members in the respective departments throughout the study period.

Ethical clearance for the primary study was obtained from ethical clearance committee at International Medical and Technological University (IMTU). Permission at referral facilities was sought from offices of municipal medical officers of health and facility in-charges of each hospital. Participants were approached with a verbal informed consent prior to recruitment into the primary study.

3. Results

We successfully analysed 40981 women-hours of follow-up. They consisted of all patients who underwent Total Abdominal Hysterectomy at Amana, Mwananyamala and Temeke regional referral hospitals from March to October 2017. In essence, none of the patient seroconverted against HIV during follow-up period, making an HIV-incidence of 0/40981 patient-hours. Their pre-operative HIV-serostata included 19 (17.76%) who were *reactive* on both screening tests, thereby considered as seropositive for HIV anti-IgG; 84 (78.5%) *non-reactive* on both screening tests and considered seronegative for HIV anti-IgG. Moreover, 3 (2.8%) patients refused screening. Therefore, their HIV-serostata remained unknown to study investigators. Likewise, 1 (0.93%) patient had discordant results between the two screening tests. All efforts to determine her HIV-serostatus during the time of hospital stay were deemed unsuccessful. All studied patients were black Africans by origin. The median age was 42 (IQR: 37.5–47) years. Serial correlation between HIV-serostata and age of patients yielded statistically significant findings ($\gamma = -0.514$, $P < 0.001$). **Figure 1** below highlights the pattern of the observed serial correlation between chronological age and HIV-serostata of participants.

To test for potential confounding, other variables (i.e. +/− of comorbidities, reported recent (past 1-month) sexual (oral, vaginal/anal) history, 1-month prior blood -(products) transfusion episode and place of residence) were also tested but yielded non-significant statistical evidence of confounding (χ^2-Yates corrected = 0.3833, df = 3). Converesely, it is worth noting that we also found a just significant correlation between reported marital and HIV stata (see **Tables 1** and **2** below) on univariate analysis during initial data exploration.

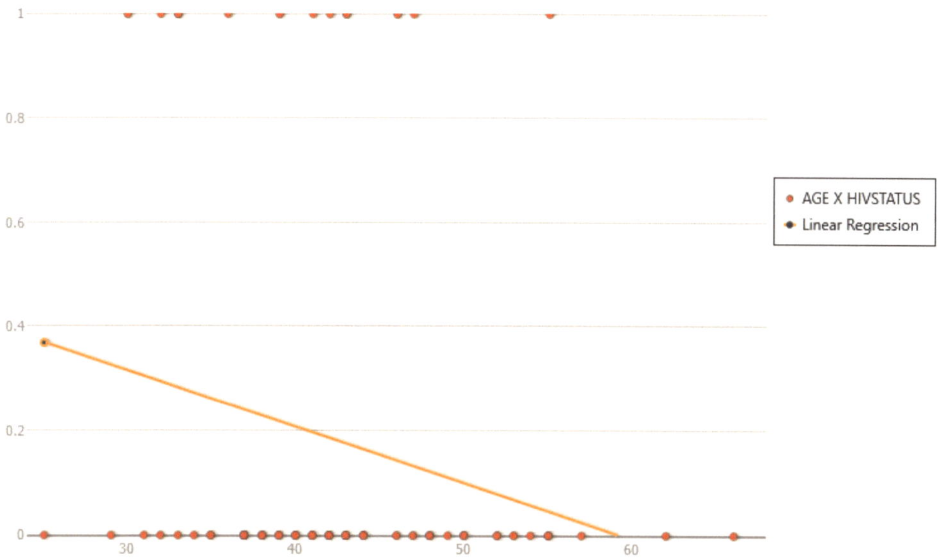

Figure 1.
Serial correlation between HIV serostata and age among women who underwent total abdominal hysterectomy in Dar es Salaam regional referral hospitals, Tanzania (March–October 2017).

HIV serostatus	Single	Married	Widowed	Divorced	Total
HIV seropositive	3	11	0	5	19
HIV seronegative	9	60	9	6	84
Total	12	71	9	11	103[1]

NOTE: *Cochran–Mantel-Hanzel corrected* χ^2 *value for the association = 8.0176, df = 3.*
[1]N = 107 but 3 individuals refused HIV screening and 1 had discordant HIV results.

Table 1.
Distribution of HIV by marital stata among women who underwent total abdominal hysterectomy in Dar es Salaam regional referral hospitals, Tanzania (March-October 2017).

Variable	Estimates	95% C.I.
Age*	- 0.8156	- 0.7488–0.9970
Marital status**	1.6429	1.3914–1.9216
Intercept	0.449	***

N.B.: *The model fitness was deemed desirable with LR value of 8.1142 and df = 2.*
**Age was coded in a binary fashion with the cut-off of 45 years (average time for natural menopause?) and found to attain linearity with the logit function. Thus, Age < 45 was used as a reference group.*
***Marital status was collapsed to married/non-married in order to attain model specification of linearity with the logit function. Here, non-married was the reference group.*

Table 2.
Findings on the multivariable logistic regression analysis of HIV-stata on ageing among women who underwent total abdominal hysterectomy in Dar es Salaam regional referral hospitals, Tanzania (March-October 2017).

4. Discussion

We detected *a statistically significant association for the probable drop in HIV-risk after age of 45 among hysterectomised women*. The finding translates to an average drop of about 30% in HIV-risk for each annual increase in life expectancy after the age of 45 years. From an evolutionary perspective, our findings are likely to be a reflection of *antagonistic pleiotropy* theory of ageing. It is evident in literature as part of a non-adaptive evolution of ageing process, as per reproductive senescence assumption. However, a word of caution - *it was a statistical estimate, out of secondary data analysis!* We therefore in a pioneering move, call for biologically plausible prospective study designs, to substantiate the exact cause of our current observed statistical puzzle!

By reflecting the nature of our target population, we derived *a possibility for hormonal interplay that potentiate HIV-entry in women during their reproductive age; and significantly drop upon cessation of menses or removal of their endocrine uteri*. Several studies in the past have suggested potential roles of female reproductive hormones in facilitating HI-viral entry and proliferation in female epithelial tissues [22–27]. For instance, Aaron Weinberg and his colleagues showed for the 1st time back in 2003, that HIV-1 induced β-defensin expression in human *oral epithelial cells, with subsequent HIV-1 replication blockage, by the β-defensin 2 & 3, via direct interaction with virions, and also through modulation of CXCR4-tropic* HIV-1 isolates [24]. To our views, Weinsberg's findings were novel even though the target was oral (rather than genital) epithelia [24]. Likewise, Morrison and colleagues performed an individual data 18-prospective studies incorporating 2-stages random effect meta-analysis with 43613 women-years of follow-up, that resulted to an adjusted Hazard Ratio (aHR) of 1.5 (95% C.I.: 1.24-1.86) upon usage of Depot Medroxyprogesterone Acetate (DMPA) [22]. Morrison study controlled for incident known biological and behavioural risk factors [22]. Progesterone (and not oestradiol) was associated with increased risks in those studies [22, 23, 26, 27]. However, causality has not been established on this topic. We hope our study findings have added quantitative estimates of association between HIV and ageing endocrine processes in non-gravid female humans.

The estimated HIV burden (17.76%) reported in our study is higher than recently reported HIV/AIDS statistics in Tanzanian general population. Tanzania's HIV Impact Survey 2016–2017 reported HIV prevalence of 6.5% among women aged 15–64 years [28]. However, our study population was unlikely to be representative of all women in Tanzania. Another contrasting factor was our limited time of follow-up, in days rather than months or years, normally applied for HIV-seroconversion incidence studies. The zero incidence in HIV-seroconversion rate observed may also likely be a function of limited time of follow-up. Moreover, of special interest to our findings, was the link between removal of endocrine uterus (a marker of *ageing* process) and HIV-risk. On average, a linear association accounted for more than half the variation between HIV-risk and chronological age. Besides, the negative sign in the correlation estimate; signified a probable reduction in HIV-risk with increasing age. It was additional statistical evidence, besides the estimated odds ratio statistic found on the linear model. However, we wish to caution against potentiality for both Berkson's and ecological fallacies when generalizing our findings. We wish our findings to be taken as *a treasure hunt* rather than justifiable evidence at present. For instance, we see a *potential for malice*, upon generalisation of these findings at individual level. We wish to caution readers, that the statistics on reduction in HIV-risk with ageing was analysed at group level. Otherwise, the same finding has several alternative explanations.

First, although the current analysis involved all women who underwent hysterectomies during the study period, and hence the estimate unlikely to be due to sampling variability, we did not have a control group by design. Moreover, there was relatively fewer individuals, in old age (>65 years) category. The analysis was therefore under-powered for detection of the observation among *senior citizens* per se. Middle aged women constituted the majority in our study population. The young and middle age groups are evident to be the most affected by HIV in Tanzania [28]. However, that evidence is doubted in present day Tanzania [29], as HIV has achieved a stable chronic status at community level. Historical data on predominance of young/middle aged members on HIV statistics in Tanzania by their own do not rule out high HIV incidence/prevalence in old aged group. Thus, it is equally likely, that our current findings to be a *statistical artifact* than a real phenomenon. However, the fact that even with the notable *under-powered statistics*, the observation was still statistically significant; is worth *speculations* towards a probable real biological phenomenon. The view follows a common knowledge, that it is relatively difficult to attain statistical significance in under-powered dataset than adequately (over)- powered dataset. We therefore strongly call for biological and clinical research on this specific topic.

Likewise, Tanzania just like other sub-Sahara African countries has never included ≥ 65 years cohort in its national HIV/AIDS surveys. This is for a variety of reasons including assumption of HIV-infection as a disease of youth and young adults. That assumption is considered by authors as a complete myth at present. The reason for disputing that assumption as a myth has been published before [29]. Otherwise, data on HIV-statistics among ≥ 65 years in Tanzania are scanty. Of the few available ones, there is one with evidence that reported a *relatively* low point prevalence (2.1%) [30].

It constituted senior community-dwelling females in North-Eastern Tanzania [30]. Currently, we are hesitant to assume that single retrieved community prevalence study to be nationally representative. Given the obvious gap, it is naturally justified that further population-based studies are needed on this topic.

Moreover, there is a specific call for interventions targeting ageing process, and senior citizens morbid and mortal statistics the world over, to be derived from reliable and valid tools. For instance, there is growing evidence that most scales and indicators used for assessing senior citizens morbid conditions report indices with questionable reliability globally [31]. One member of our team has just published his findings [31], that showed the current global scales and indicators for assessing frailty to record reliability values that were lower than *greatest lower bound* (*glb*) reliability estimate [31]. Part of the challenge has been contributed by years-long tendency of editors and reviewers to consider Chronbach's alpha coefficient as *a sin qua non* for defining reliability index in scientific literature. We could not control all biases associated with our quantitative variables nor did we assume perfection in the literature cited in this chapter, against all systematic and measurement errors in them. The fact that the world is ageing fast, especially sub-Sahara African countries [32], calls for tools with appreciable precision and accuracy during data collection & reporting processes. Thus, studies on biological, clinical, public health, demographic as well as economic analyses of ageing processes are highly warranted globally. Our message given the current statistical findings, *some somatic maintenance properties are likely to be retained (reversed) after reproductive years in female humans!*

Likewise, we took a careful measure not to overlook the finding on HIV and marital stata. There was a rather strong ego to consider that finding as spurious, but indeed the decision was not supported by a logical flow of reasoning among investigators. In fact, we are still debating! Previous studies in similar settings yielded confusing results [33–35], with one study from a population based study in Tanzania that conferred an almost additional 50% risk (aOR: 1.49, 95% C.I.: 1.08–2.04) to remarried couples compared to single/cohabiting partners [35]. Otherwise, the fact that HIV-infection has been present in Tanzania since 1983 [29], and ante-retro viral drugs against HIV became available in mid-1990's [29]; justifies possibilities for residual vertical infection, among infants born with HIV from infected parent(s), to proceed to adulthood. Should this speculation be valid, assumptions related to exclusively acquired HIV risks after sexual maturity could be nullified. Evidently, a member of our research group once co-authored a population based study, among under-fives in a sub-urb of Tanzania, that realized potential sources of infectious ailments, via a domain of febrile illnesses [36]. However, details about the HIV-associated behavioural risks as well as impact of Ante-Retro-Viral drugs against HIV to babies born with the disease were beyond the objective of our current and previous works. Thus, we do believe there is a desperate need for future studies on the mechanisms behind preponderance of HIV infection among participants who reported in married category.

Lastly, much as we do believe our current findings to be reflective of antagonistic pleiotropy theory of ageing process, we wish to address some other important limitations of our findings. It has been a general consensus that women tend to outlive men in longevity studies [37–42]. Even though most scholars of the past (and likely the present?) still associate the reason(s) back to environmental causes [42]; there is a clear indication, that the concept to have an underlying biological and/or clinical causes [37–41]. Mysteriously to our current findings, there have been previous studies that reported female advantages in HIV-survival patterns whether or not on anteretroviral treatment in similar settings [43, 44]. Thus, female survival advantages tend to manifest both against HIV-risks as well as in HIV-infection whether or not the latter factor is associated with treatment. Besides, we could not set up an enough time follow-up study in order to arrive with our current conclusion. However, we do believe what we just showed (probably for the first time?) to the world to be an otherwise real biological phenomenon, that has been part of knowledge base in what is currently referred to as biogerontology.

5. Conclusions

There was an observed statistically significant reduced risk of HIV with ageing process in this secondary analysis. None of the studied women seroconverted against HIV during our follow-up period. Point prevalence of HIV among total hysterectomised women was higher than otherwise reported in the Tanzania's general population. Patients reported to be married had a statistically significant higher chance of being HIV-seropositive than others in this study population.

Acknowledgements

We express sincere votes of thanks to the management of the International Medical & Technological University (IMTU) for guidance and promotion of this research activity. We also aknowledge I-Katch technology Ltd through its *Coffeeshop clinical research & scientific writing programme*. Moreover, we hereby express our thanking note to Café aroma in Dar es Salaam, Tanzania. Café aroma provided a near perfect environment (coffee, free-wifi and wonderful caloric-burning standing office tables) through which most of our meetings during study research question formulation, early study designs and data analysis were done, at times in their busiest business hours. *Dr Godfrey Ruben Swai* of The Registered Trustees of Ultimate Family Healthcare in Dar es salaam, Tanzania is credited for timely peer review, and insightful opinion on the quality of the final draft. Lastly but most important, we wish to eternally recognize the willingness of all women who consented wholeheartedly to be part of the primary study.

Conflict of interest

The authors declare no conflict of interest.

Author details

Kelvin Leshabari[1,2*], Godfrey Chale[2,3] and Rashid Salim[3]

1 Ageing Research Group, Registered Trustees of Ultimate Family Healthcare, Dar es Salaam, Tanzania

2 Clinical Research Unit, I-Katch Technology Ltd, Dar es Salaam, Tanzania

3 Department of Obstetrics and Gynaecology, International Medical and Technological University, Dar es Salaam, Tanzania

*Address all correspondence to: kelvin@familyhealth.or.tz; celsius_lx@yahoo.co.uk

References

[1] Klein S, Flanagan K. Sex differences in immune responses. Nature Reviews Immunology. 2016;**16**:626-638

[2] Kiess W, Belohradsky B. Endocrine regulation of the immune system. Klinische Wochenschrift. 1986;**64**:1-7

[3] Stelzer I, Arck P. Immunity and the endocrine system. Encyclopedia of Immunobiology. 2016:73-85

[4] Beagley K, Gockel C. Regulation of innate and adaptive immunity by the female sex hormones oestradiol and progesterone. FEMS Immunology & Medical Microbiology. 2003;**38**(1):13-22

[5] Wessels J, Felker A, Dupont H, Kaushic C. The relationship between sex hormones, the vaginal microbiome and immunity in HIV-1 susceptibility in women. Disease Models & Mechanisms. 2018;**11**(9):dmm 035147. DOI: 10.1242/dmm.035147

[6] Polis C, Curtis K, Hannaford P, Phillips S, Chipato T, Kiarie J, et al. An updated systematic review of epidemiological evidence on hormonal contraceptive methods and HIV acquisition in women. AIDS. 2016;**30**: 2665-2683

[7] King A, Critchley H, Kelley R. Innate immune defences in the human endometrium. Reproductive Biology and Endocrinology. 2003;**1**:116

[8] McIntyre R, Hunt J. Antigen presenting cells and HLA-GL a review. Placenta. 2005;**26**(suppl. A):S104-S109

[9] Dulioust E, Du A, Costagliola D, Guibert J, Kunstmann J, Heard I, et al. Semen alterations in HIV-1 infected men. Human Reproduction. 2002;**17**(8): 2112-2118

[10] Toumala R, Kalish L, Zorilla C, Fox H, Shearer W, Landay A, et al. Changes in total, CD4+ and CD8+ lymphocytes during pregnancy and 1-year postpartum in human immunodeficiency virus-infected women. The women and infants transmission study. Obstetrics and Gynecology. 1997;**89**(6):667-674

[11] Sheffield J, Wendel G Jr, McIntyre D, Norgard M. The effect of progesterone levels and pregnancy on HIV-1 coreceptor expression. Reproductive Sciences. 2009;**16**:20-31

[12] Kourtis A, Read J, Jamieson D. Pregnancy and infection. The New England Journal of Medicine. 2014;**370**: 2211-2218

[13] Marston M, Newell M, Crampin A, Lutalo T, Musoke R, Gregson S, et al. Is the risk of HIV acquisition increased during and immediately after pregnancy? A secondary analysis of pooled HIV community-based studies from the ALPHA network. PLoS One. 2013;**8**(12): e82219

[14] Morrison C, Wang J, Van der Pol B, Padian N, Salata R, Richardson B. Pregnancy and the risk of HIV-1 acquisition among women in Uganda and Zimbabwe. AIDS. 2007;**21**(8):1027-1034

[15] Thompson K, Hughes J, Baeten J, John-Stewart G, Celum C, Cohen C, et al. Increased risk of HIV acquisition among women throughout pregnancy and during postpartum period: A prospective per-coital-act analysis among women with HIV-infected partners. The Journal of Infectious Diseases. 2018;**218**:16-25

[16] Mitchell C, Hitti J, Paul K, Agnew K, Cohn S, Luque A, et al. Cervicovaginal shedding of HIV type 1 is related to

genital tract inflammation independent of changes in vaginal microbiota. AIDS Research and Human Retroviruses. 2011; **27**(1):35-39

[17] Phoswa W. The role of HIV infection in the pathophysiology of gestational diabetes mellitus and hypertensive disorders of pregnancy. Frontiers in Cardiovascular Medicine. 2021;**8**:613930

[18] Gillespie S, Porter K, Christian L. Adaptation of the inflammatory immune response across pregnancy and postpartum in black and white women. Journal of Reproductive Immunology. 2016;**114**:27-31

[19] Turner L, Shepherd J, Wang L, Bunker C, Lowder J. Hysterectomy surgery trends: A more accurate depiction of the last decade? American Journal of Obstetrics and Gynecology. 2013;**208**(4):277e1-277e7

[20] Oliphant S, Jones K, Wang L, Bunker C, Lowder J. Trends over time with commonly performed obstetric and gynecologic inpatients procedures. Obstetrics and Gynecology. 2010;**116**(4): 926-931

[21] Kasiulevicius V, Sapoka V, Filipavisiute R. Sample size calculation in epidemiological studies. Gerontology 2006;**7**:225-231

[22] Morrison C, Chen P-L, Kwok C, Baeten J, Brown J, Crook A, et al. Hormonal contraceptions and the risk of HIV acquisition: An individual participant data meta-analysis. PLoS Medicine. 2015;**12**(1):e1001778

[23] Happigold J, Kaushic C, Hel Z. Hormonal contraceptions and HIV-1 acquisition: Biological mechanisms. Endocrine Reviews. 2018;**39**:36-78

[24] Quinones-Mateu M, Lederman M, Feng Z, Chakraborty B, Weber J, Rangel H, et al. Human epithelial β-defensins 2 and 3 inhibit HIV-1 replication. AIDS. 2003;**17**(16):F39-F48

[25] Pioli P, Weaver L, Schaefer T, Wright J, Wira C, Guyre P. Lipopolysaccharide-induced IL-1β production by human uterine macrophages up-regulates uterine epithelial cells expressions of human β-defensins 2. The Journal of Immunology. 2006;**176**:6647-6655

[26] Pioli P, Jensen A, Weaver L, Amiel E, Shen Z, Shen L, et al. Oestradiol attenuates lipopolysaccharide-induced CXC chemokine ligand 8 production by human peripheral blood monocytes. Journal of Immunology. 2007;**179**: 6284-6290

[27] Byrne E, Anahtar M, Cohen K, Moodley A, Padavattan N, Ismail N, et al. Association between injectable progestin only contraceptives and HIV acquisition and HIV target cell frequency in the female genital tract in south African women: A prospective cohort study. The Lancet Infectious Diseases. 2016;**16**(4):441-448

[28] Tanzania HIV Impact Survey (THIS) 2016–2017. Available from: http://www.nbs.go.tz/nbs/takwimu/this201617/Tanzania_SummarySheet_English.pdf, 2018 [Accessed: 10 January 2022]

[29] Leshabari K, Ashok K, Gebuis E, Leshabari S, Ohnishi M. Challenges in morbidity and mortality statistics of the elderly population in Tanzania: A call to action. Quality in Ageing & Older Adults. 2017;**18**(3):171-174

[30] Swai S, Damian D, Urassa S, Temba B, Mahande M, Philemon R, et al. Prevalence and risk factors for HIV among people aged 50 years and older in Rombo district, northern Tanzania.

Tanzania Journal of Health Research. 2017;**19**(2):1-6. Available from: https://www.ajol.info/index.php/thrb/article/viewFile/147510/144522 [Accessed: 10 January 2022]

[31] Leshabari K. Reliability and validity of clinico-pathological features associated with frailty syndrome in elderly population. In: Palermo S, editor. Frailty in the Elderly – Understanding and Managing Complexities. London: Intech Open; 2021. DOI: 10.5772/intechopen.93499. Available from: https://www.intechopen.com/chapters/73143 [Accessed: 5 August 2021]

[32] Leshabari K. Demographic transition in sub-Saharan Africa: From grassroots to ivory towers. In: Klimczuk A, editor. Demographic Analysis – Selected Concepts, Tools and Applications. London: IntechOpen; 2021. DOI: 10.5772/intechopen.98407. Available from: https://www.intechopen.com/chapters/77806 [Accessed: 1 January 2022]

[33] Shisana O, Risher K, Celentano D, Zungu N, Rehle T, Ngcaweni B, et al. Does marital status matter in an HIV hyperendemic country? Findings from 2012 South African National HIV prevalence, incidence and behaviour survey. AIDS Care. 2016;**28**(2): 234-241

[34] Shisana O, Zungu-Dirwayi N, Toefy Y, Simbayi L, Malik S, Zuma K. Marital status and risk of HIV infection in South Africa. South African Medical Journal. 2004;**94**:537-543

[35] Mtenga S, Pfeiffer C, Merten S, Mamdani M, Exavery A, Haafkens J, et al. Prevalence and social drivers of HIV among married and cohabitating heterosexual adults in south-eastern Tanzania: analysis of adult health community cohort data. Global Health Action. 2015;**8**. DOI: 10.3402/gha.v8.28941

[36] Leshabari K, Ramji R. The pattern of infection among under-fives: a call for actions. Dar es Salaam Medical Students' Journal. 2008;**15**(1): 24-28

[37] Lang E, Arnold K, Kupfer P. [Women live longer–biological, medical and sociological causes] Z Gerontol. 1994;**27**(1):10-15

[38] Stindl R. Tying it all together: telomeres, sexual size dimorphism and the gender gap in life expectancy. Medical Hypotheses. 2004;**62**:151-154

[39] Biecek P, Cebrat S. Why Y-chromosome is shorter and women live longer? European Physical Journal B. 2008;**65**:149-153

[40] Ginter E, Simko V. Women live longer than men. Bratisl Lek Listy. 2013; **114**(02):45-49

[41] Goldin C, lleras-Muney A. XX > XY?: The changing female advantages in life expectancy. NEBR Working paper No. 24716, 2018. Available from: https://www.nber.org/papers/w24716 [Accessed: 1 January 2022]

[42] Austad S. Why women live longer than men: sex differences in longevity. Gender Medicine. 2006;**3**(2):79-92

[43] Taylor-Smith K, Tweya H, Harries A, Schoutene E, Jahn A. Gender differences in retention and survival on anteretroviral therapy of HIV-1 infected adults in Malawi. Malawi Medical Journal. 2010;**22**(2):49-56

[44] Dovel K, Yeatman S, Watkins S, Poulin M. Men's heightened risk of AIDS-related death: the legacy of gendered HIV testing and treatment strategies. AIDS. 2015;**29**(10):1123-1125

Chapter 9

The Role of IL-6 in RNA Virus Infection

Rizaldy Taslim Pinzon

Abstract

IL-6 is a pleiotropic cytokine produced in response to tissue damage and infections. This up-regulation was observed during infection with a highly virulent VSV strain. There was potential association between IL-6 levels and virus virulence. In this chapter we would like to explore in more detail the biological functions of IL-6 in different virus models. We also discuss the debatable role of IL-6 during viral infections. Previous studies show the potential role of IL-6 to mount a proper immune response during some viral infections, others link this cytokine with exacerbation of viral disease. These latter findings lend support to the hypothesis that up-regulation of IL-6 during certain viral infections may promote virus survival and/or exacerbation of clinical disease. Previous experimental evidences also suggest potential negative consequences that increased levels of IL-6 might have on the cellular immune response against viruses.

Keywords: RNA virus-IL6-soluble-imune-host

1. Introduction

The pandemic of coronavirus disease 2019 (COVID-19) caused by severe acute respiratory syndrome coronavirus 2 (SARS-CoV-2) has set a major healthcare issues and economic burden worldwide. Like other RNA viruses, SARS-CoV-2, while adapting to their new human hosts, is prone to genetic evolution with the development of mutations over time, resulting in mutant variants that may have different characteristics than its ancestral strains. Currently, treatments of COVID-19 are mainly repurposing drugs or symptomatic with no definitive treatment directed against the virus [1].

Coronaviruses (CoVs), enveloped positive-sense RNA viruses, are characterized by club-like spikes that project from their surface, an unusually large RNA genome, and a unique replication strategy. In the absence of specific treatment or antiviral drugs been proven against SARS-CoV-2, researchers have proposed many therapeutics agents used as adjunctive treatments for COVID-19 patients apart from supplemental oxygen therapy or mechanical ventilation [1, 2].

In Coronavirus infection, viral surface glycoproteins, double-stranded RNA, and intracellular viral proteins all have the capacity to activate signal transduction pathways leading to the expression of cytokines and chemokines. Cytokine storm is one of the main mechanisms of the disease and is believed to trigger an exaggerated immune response in the host and has been observed more frequently in severe COVID-19 patients associated with complications, such as acute respiratory distress syndrome (ARDS) and other multiple organ injuries [2].

An important consequence of RNA virus infection and COVID-19 disease is cell-free DNA (cfDNA) found in body fluids such as serum or plasma. cfDNA originates from nuclear or mitochondrial DNA released from dead/dying cells, DNA released from live cells, and foreign DNA from invading viruses [3]. The other interesting points are the fact that monoclonal antibody against IL-6 receptors or IL-6 inhibitor has shown to be an effective agent in COVID-19 patients with severe illness. Initially, it is frequently used for the treatment of rheumatoid arthritis patients. These drugs targeting IL-6 as inflammatory mediators will decrease inflammatory response in cytokine storm, hence minimizing the incidence of jeopardize complications, such as ARDS. Tocilizumab and other anti-IL-6 receptors antagonist has been recommended as an immunotherapy in severely ill patients and improved the clinical outcomes as well as decrease in mortality rate [3, 4]. The aim of this review is describe the role of IL-6 in RNA virus infection.

2. Method

This article is a narrative review study include IL-6 and RNA virology, clinical impact, diagnosis, and treatment. The search was conducted using five keywords "IL-6," "RNA Virus," "IL-6 inhibitors" in combination with "human" in PubMed, Scopus, and ScienceDirect among articles between 2000 and April 2022. We focused on publications post-year 2000, with emphasis on the past 10 years, but we did not exclude commonly referenced, relevant, and influential older publications. The clinical trial, case–control, review, and a meta-analysis study of 20 years; 2000–2022 articles, case series, cohort, and cross-sectional studies were reviewed. We also reviewed the references of each article to include further other studies or reports not identified by the search. We excluded articles considering the expert viewpoints and letters to the editor. We limit our search to English written articles and articles on human study.

3. Discussion

3.1 Inflammatory cytokine (IL-6) and RNA virus infection

After RNA virus entered the host. The innate immune system is the first line defensive mechanism for this virus. The response will be responsible for detecting pathogen-associated molecular patterns (PAMPs). Viral RNA is a potent inducer of antiviral innate immune signaling. It will provokes an antiviral state by directing expression of interferons (IFNs) and pro-inflammatory cytokines. The +RNA viruses developed various methods to avoid detection and downstream signaling. This mechanism includes isolation of viral RNA replication in membranous viral replication organelles (ROs) [5].

The defense mechanism of the host includes rapid production interferons and other pro-inflammatory cytokines. This is an important consequence of virus detection. This condition contributes to an antiviral state in both the infected host cell and other surrounding cells. The next phases showed that interferons will play an essential role in coordinating the antiviral adaptive response system [5].

One of the most studied cytokines is IL-6. In RNA virus infection IL-6 is considered one of the most important cytokines during an infection, along with interleukin 1 (IL-1) and tumor necrosis factor alpha (TNF-a). IL-6 is a pleotropic cytokine produced in response many types of tissue damage including fibroblasts, keratinocytes, mesangial cells, vascular endothelial cells, mast cells, macrophages, dendritic cells, and T and B cells. After targeting its specific receptor, IL-6 starts a cascade of signaling events mainly associated with the JAK/STAT3 (Janus kinase (JAK)/signal transducer and activator of transcription 3) activation pathway. This cascade will promote the transcription of multiple downstream genes associated with cellular signaling processes, including cytokines, receptors, adaptor proteins, and protein kinases. It will also regulate the production of proteins implicated in regulation of many gene expression. The biological consequences of IL-6 production have been associated with pro inflammatory effects [5, 6].

As an immediate answer after RNA virus infections, different immune cellular pathogen recognition receptors, including toll-like receptors (TLR:2, 3, 4, 7, 8, and 9), nucleotide-binding oligomerization domain-like receptors, and retinoic acid-inducible gene-1-like receptors, are able to sense a variety of pathogen-associated molecular patterns displayed by viruses (envelope glycoproteins, single and double-stranded RNA), which stimulate transcription of IL-6 among other proinflammatory cytokines [5].

IL-6 play significant role either in positive or negative ways. The animal studies showed its ability to repress the replication of CSFV (classical swine fever virus) in swine peripheral blood mononuclear cells. However, experimental scientific evidence also suggests the negative impact of increasing IL-6 level. The potential role of IL-6 increase is the establishment of a viral persistent state in infected hosts. The animal studies showed that overexpression of IL-6 during the viral immune response might induce viral persistence by impairing the polarization and functionality of Th1 cells and the lytic capacity of CD8 T-cells through different mechanisms, leading to chronic infections. As a consequence of the constant antigen stimulation, CD8 T-cells become unresponsive and fail to develop into memory CD8 T-cells, a situation that limits viral clearance. The other negative impact of upregulated IL-6 is increasing inflammation followed by cytokine secretion and cellular recruitment as described during autoimmune diseases. This inflammation state may be an advantage for some RNA viruses by providing new targets for subsequent infections [6, 7].

Previous report and reviews showed that high levels of interleukin 6 (IL-6) and Interleukin 8 (IL 8) were found in the very acute stage associated with lung lesions in SARS-CoV-1 patients. The IL-6 can induce the hyper-innate inflammatory response. In the cases of SARS-CoV-1, very high levels of IL-6 were associated with significant and severe inflammation state, and its correlated with high mortality. Some observational retrospective and systematic review/meta-analysis showed that high IL-6 and C-reactive protein (CRP) were significantly correlate with mortality and severity of the disease. Some recent evidences also proved that critically ill patients with severe respiratory failure and SARS-CoV-2 have either immune dysregulation or macrophage-activation syndrome, both of which are characterized by pro-inflammatory cytokines (IL-6). The immune dysregulation, in particular, is driven by the Interleukin-6 (IL-6). The most significant impact of this condition features of this immune dysregulation are: (1) over-production of pro-inflammatory cytokines by monocytes, and (2) lymphocyte dysregulation with CD4 lymphopenia [7, 8].

After the pandemic of COVID-19, some recent evidences showed that there are of many similarities between Macrophage Activation Syndrome (MAS) disease and

COVID-19 pneumonia. This phenomenon is a pathological condition that called over production of cytokine secretion. The loss of first line anti-viral defense mechanism may be responsible for this activation. It will cause prolonging and sustained IL-6 secretion. The Sustained IL-6 secretion was also correlated with the serum viral RNA load [7–9].

3.2 The up regulation of IL-6 in RNA virus infection

In common, pathogen-associated molecular patterns (PAMPs) recognized by pathogen recognition receptors (PRRs) in RNA virus infected lesions. The damage-associated molecular patterns (DAMPs) released from damaged cells in non-infectious inflammation will provoke IL-6 synthesis in many cells such as immune-competent cells, mesenchymal cells, fibroblasts, endothelial cells, and epithelial cells [10, 11]. The IL-6 initiates warning signals to the entire body, and many experiments have shown that serum IL-6 levels are elevated in patients RNA virus infection. Some studies in Hepatitis B virus infection showed that IL-6 is also a good marker for HBV-related disease progression [12]. The levels of IL-6 are significantly higher in chronic hepatitis B (CHB) patients than in healthy individuals [13]. The IL-6 is also significantly higher in patients with advanced liver disease (LC or HCC) compared to the CHB groups [14].

The IL-6 is an important proinflammatory cytokines during RNA virus infection onset, especially, at the mucosal sites. However, the impact of IL-6 on the disease outcome may vary significantly. The IL-6-dependent Th17 activation and differentiation are important for effective neutrophil migration, IL-6 together with IL-15 modulate cytolytic capacity of $CD8^+$ T cells [15]. In this part, IL-6, as a pyrogenic cytokine, contributes to thermostatic regulation that is very important for effective anti-viral response [16].

On the other hand, the upregulation of IL-6 has been implicated in the progression of RNA viral infections. In this part, IL-6 synergizes with IL-1b and TNF to upregulate trypsin expression, trypsin activates matrix metalloproteinases and causes the breakdown of basal membrane and extracellular matrix, that cause increased tissue permeability and edema [17]. The upregulation of IL-6 promotes Th17 cell differentiation and IL-17A secretion, which, in turn, activates the expression of anti-apoptotic molecules, such as Bcl-X_L, favoring survival of virus-infected cells in the model of persistent viral infection [18]. In the COVID-19 infection, the increase of IL-17 that mediated by IL-6 promotes the migration of neutrophils whichcontribute to the pathogenesis of ARDS [19, 20].

- IL-6 promotes highly specific reaction of adaptive immunity by stimulating of $CD8^+$ T cells and B cells, which is balanced by T regulatory cells.

- IL-6 facilitates survival of phagocytic neutrophils.

- IL-6 can provide unfavorable Th2 and Th17 over Th1 helper differentiation and facilitate tissue injury by dysregulation of extracellular matrix and attraction of neutrophils and pro-inflammatory macrophages (**Figure 1**).

3.3 Clinical implication

What are the implications of this findings? There is a fact that some viral strains can cross the barrier of the immune response and induce the over-production of IL-6. This condition correlated with the advancement of viral activity. This

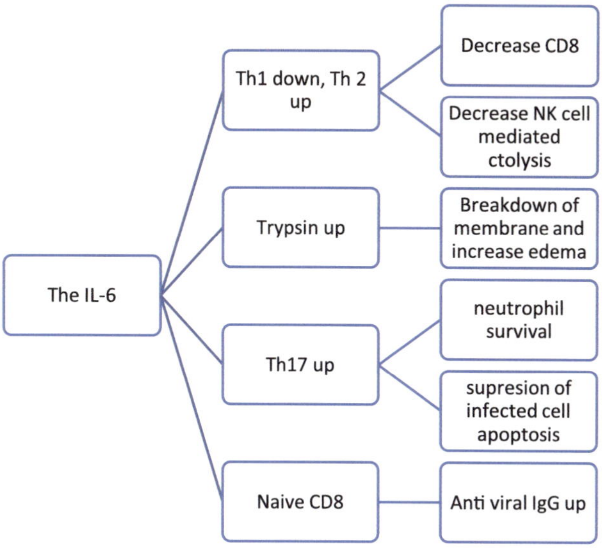

Figure 1.
The IL-6 demonstrates opposing effects during the immune response to viral infections [6].

condition consequently followed by an up-regulation in the production of IL-6, this polymorphisms in the region of the IL-6 gene stimulate the overexpression of IL-6 that also correlated with viral progression. This loop correlated with the increase of the viruses virulence that damaging Th1 cell polarization and functionality. This condition caused viremia and the loss of CD8 T-cells ability to develop memory cells, thus reducing the capacity to fight viral load. Constant replication of the virus fails to grow into long-out plasma cells, limiting their ability to clear the virus Prolonged RNA virus infections increase levels of IL-6, that further makes accumulation of this pathologies state (inflammation plus cytokines and cellular presence). This state may be advantageous for several RNA viruses, mainly because it offers some opportunities for near-future infections because there are new target cells to choose from. There were a debate on how is the inflammatory cytokine, IL-6, in viral infections can be used as a biomarker for prognosis. An exploration of the IL-6 function as well as that of IL-6 inhibition in treating persistent infections might aid in developing its therapeutic benefit may reveal information about its utility [8, 9].

The study from Saji et al. showed that IL-6 is important prognosis biomarker. The study from 102 patients with moderate to severe COVID-19 showed that the 30-day was significantly higher in patients with high IL-6 (> 49 pg./mL) and SARS-CoV-2 RNAaemia (> 1.5 copies/μL) compared to those with high IL-6 or RNAaemia or without high IL-6 and RNAaemia (88% vs. 22% or 8%, *log-rank test* $P = 0.0097$ or $P < 0.0001$, respectively) [17].

The other study in showed similar result. Patients with hypoxemia had significantly higher concentrations of IL-6, C-reactive protein, procalcitonin, fibrinogen, total bilirubin, aspartate aminotransferase and alanine aminotransferase at initial screening. ROC analyses identified IL-6 as the most robust predictor of hypoxemia. The concentration of IL-6 > 24 pg./mL predicted the development of hypoxemia with the sensitivity of 100% and specificity of 88.9%. The positive and negative predictive values were 76.9, and 100% respectively [18].

The prognostic value of clinical severity also been showed. The study in the 140 COVID-19 patients, the levels of IL-6, CRP, and PCT increased in 95 (67.9%), 91 (65.0%), and 8 (5.7%) patients on admission, respectively. The proportion of patients with increased IL-6, CRP, and PCT levels was significantly higher in the severe patients than in the mild one. Cox proportional hazard model showed that IL-6 and CRP could be used as independent factors to predict the severity of COVID-19. Furthermore, patients with IL-6 > 32.1 pg./mL or CRP > 41.8 mg/L were more likely to have severe complications [19].

3.4 IL-6 inhibitor as promising treatment

IL-6 is produced by dendritic cells, macrophages, mast cells, and other innate immune cells. Several previous studies showed that IL-6 has long been considered a marker of inflammation. The increased levels of IL-6 significantly noted in number of diseases that related with ongoing inflammatory cell activation. The IL-6 can also be produced by non-immune cells such as epithelial cells, endothelial cells, keratinocytes, and fibroblasts among others, in response to specific stimuli [4].

The presence of IL-6 may not necessarily correlate with the production of other inflammatory cytokines and it may not be just a marker of ongoing inflammation, but a direct player in the immune response. A number of studies have shown a role of IL-6 in the adaptive immune response, primarily on the differentiation fate of CD4 T cells, but IL-6 can also modulate aspects of the innate immune response [17, 18].

Elevated levels of IL-6 in the lung and in serum have been found in patients infected with the influenza virus, including the 2009 H1N1 pandemic influenza [21, 22]. IL-6- and IL-6-mediated signals are essential for survival to a non-lethal dose of influenza H1N1 virus infection. Deficiency of IL-6 or IL-6R prevents clearance of the H1N1 virus in association with low numbers of neutrophils present in the lungs of infected individuals. We also show that IL-6 provides survival signals to protect neutrophils from influenza virus-triggered apoptosis. Impaired virus clearance caused by the lack of IL-6 or IL-6R signals leads to emphysema-like destruction of the lung and, ultimately, death [23, 24]. Thus, IL-6 is a protective factor against primary infection with the influenza H1N1 virus by promoting the innate phase of the immune response and virus clearance (**Figure 2**) [23, 25, 26].

With coronavirus disease 2019 (Covid-19), the role of localized inflammation was evident. Patients with severe symptoms has high interleukin-6, a cytokine produced by macrophages that induces a proinflammatory response and is often elevated in patients with Covid-19. Some studies showed the benefit of IL-6 inhibitors.

The REMACAP trials, which had an adaptive design, approximately 800 patients in need of respiratory or blood-pressure support or both were randomly assigned to placebo or a single injection of an interleukin-6 receptor blocker, tocilizumab or sarilumab. The primary outcome was a composite of in-hospital death and days free of respiratory or blood-pressure support to day 21. The group receiving an interleukin-6 receptor blocker had an in-hospital mortality of 27%, as compared with 36% in the control group, and those receiving the receptor blocker had a median of 10 to 11 organ support–free days, as compared with 0 days for control [27].

Conflicting result was shown in CONVACTA trial. This randomized, controlled trial include 452 patients with Covid-19 (oxygen saturation, ≤93%) were randomly assigned in a 2:1 ratio to receive one dose of tocilizumab or placebo. The primary outcome was clinical status at day 28; mortality was a secondary outcome. The group receiving tocilizumab had a median clinical status of 1 (discharged or ready for

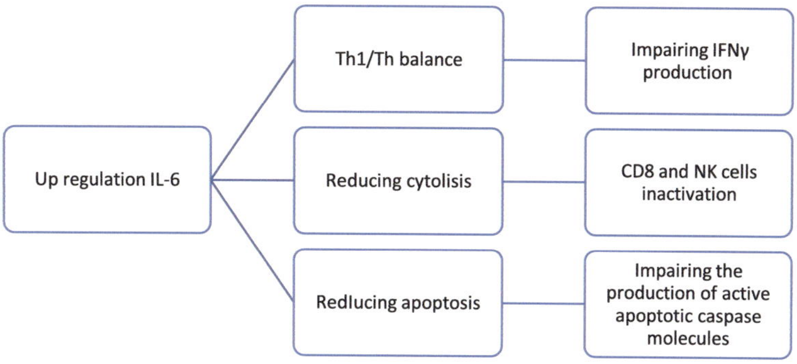

Figure 2.
Overexpression of IL6 and its negative impact [15].

discharge), and the control group had a median clinical status of 2 (out of intensive care and not receiving supplemental oxygen). Mortality was 19.7% in the tocilizumab group and 19.4% in the control group [28].

The meta-analysis of 27 randomized trials of IL-6ra that included 10,930 patients with COVID-19indicate that all-cause mortality was reduced in patients hospitalized for COVID-19 and treated with IL-6ra compared with those treated with placebo or usual care. By day 28 after randomization, 1407 deaths occurred among 6449 patients randomized to receive IL-6 antagonists and 1158 deaths occurred among 4481 patients randomized to usual care or placebo (summary odds ratio [OR], 0.86 [95% CI, 0.79–0.95]; $P = .003$ based on a fixed-effects meta-analysis). Importantly, a significant mortality benefit was only found when IL-6 inhibitor were coadministered with glucocorticoids (summary OR for the association of IL-6 antagonist treatment with 28-day all-cause mortality, 0.78 with concomitant glucocorticoid administration vs. 1.09 without glucocorticoid administration). The benefits of IL-6 inhibitor were most evident among patients who received respiratory support with oxygen by nasal cannula, face mask, high-flow nasal oxygen (OR for death, 0.81 [95% CI, 0.67–0.98]), or noninvasive ventilation (OR, 0.83 [95% CI, 0.72–0.96]) vs. those who required invasive mechanical ventilation (IMV) (OR, 0.95 [95% CI, 0.78–1.16]) [29].

The review showed that, IL-6 receptor antagonist hold promise for patients hospitalized for COVID-19 with progressive disease and substantial oxygen requirements but are not yet merited for widespread use among patients with mild disease nor with prolonged invasive mechanical ventilation [30].

4. Conclusion

There are evidences supporting a significant role of IL-6 during viral infections. IL-6 production that may be detrimental to the cellular immune response during viral infections. The change in IL-6 production during the immune response to viral infection are (i) the increased ability of some viral strains to overcome the immune response using a variety of evasion strategies, and consequently up-regulate the production of IL-6 as a result of increased viral loads, and (ii) polymorphisms in the IL-6 gene promoter stimulating overexpression of IL-6 during the immune response. The increased levels of IL-6 significantly related with ongoing inflammatory cell activation and poor prognosis.

Author details

Rizaldy Taslim Pinzon
School of Medicine, Duta Wacana Christian University, Yogyakarta, Indonesia

*Address all correspondence to: drpinzon17@gmail.com

References

[1] Yuen KS, Ye ZW, Fung SY, Chan CP, Jin DY. SARS-CoV-2 and COVID-19: The most important research questions. Cell & Bioscience. 2020;**10**:40. DOI: 10.1186/s13578-020-00404-4

[2] Mehta P, McAuley DF, Brown M, Sanchez E, Tattersall RS, Manson JJ. HLH across speciality collaboration, UK. COVID-19: Consider cytokine storm syndromes and immunosuppression. Lancet. 2020;**395**(10229):1033-1034. DOI: 10.1016/S0140-6736(20)30628-0

[3] Xu X, Han M, Li T, et al. Effective treatment of severe COVID-19 patients with tocilizumab. Proceedings of the National Academy of Sciences of the United States of America. 2020;**117**(20):10970-10975. DOI: 10.1073/pnas.2005615117

[4] Zhang C, Wu Z, Li JW, Zhao H, Wang GQ. The cytokine release syndrome (CRS) of severe COVID-19 and interleukin-6 receptor (IL-6R) antagonist tocilizumab may be the key to reduce the mortality. International Journal of Antimicrobial Agents. 2020;**55**:105954. DOI: 10.1016/j.ijantimicag.2020.105954

[5] Scutigliani EM, Kikkert K. Interaction of the innate immune system with positive-strand RNA virus replication organelles. Cytokine & Growth Factor Reviews. 2017;**37**:17-27

[6] Velazquez-Salinas L, Verdugo-Rodriguez A, Rodriguez LL, Borca MV. The role of interleukin 6 during viral infections. Frontiers in Microbiology. 2019;**10**:1057. DOI: 10.3389/fmicb.2019.01057

[7] Magro G. SARS-CoV-2 and COVID-19: Is interleukin-6 (IL-6) the 'culprit lesion' of ARDS onset? What is there besides Tocilizumab? SGP130Fc. Cytokine: X. 2020;**2**(2):100029

[8] Suliman BA. Interleukin 6 is a two-edged sword: A centerpiece in the immune response against the SARS-CoV-2. Trends in Medicine. 2021. DOI: 10.15761/TiM.1000275

[9] Malik A, Naz A, Ahmad S, Hafeez M, Awan FM, Jafar TH, et al. Inhibitory potential of phytochemicals on Interleukin-6-mediated T-cell reduction in COVID-19 patients: A computational approach. Bioinformatics and Biology Insights. 2021;**15**:11779322211021430

[10] Rose-John S. Il-6 trans-signaling via the soluble il-6 receptor: Importance for the pro-inflammatory activities of il-6. International Journal of Biological Sciences. 2012;**8**:1237-1247

[11] Tanaka T, Kishimoto T. The biology and medical implications of interleukin-6. Cancer Immunology Research. 2014;**2**:288-294

[12] Kumar H, Kawai T, Akira S. Pathogen recognition by the innate immune system. International Reviews of Immunology. 2011;**30**:16-34

[13] Zhang F, Yao S, Zhang M, Yuan J, Chen X, Zhou B. Roles of circulating soluble interleukin (il)-6 receptor and il-6 receptor expression on cd4+ t cells in patients with chronic hepatitis b. International Journal of Infectious Diseases. 2011;**15**:e267-e271

[14] Song le H, Binh VQ, Duy DN, Kun JF, Bock TC, Kremsner PG, et al. Serum cytokine profiles associated with clinical presentation in vietnamese infected with hepatitis b virus. Journal of Clinical Virology. 2003;**28**:93-103

[15] Yang R, Masters AR, Fortner KA, Champagne DP, Yanguas-Casas N, Silberger DJ, et al. IL-6 promotes the differentiation of a subset of naive CD8+ T cells into IL-21-producing B helper CD8+ T cells. The Journal of Experimental Medicine. 2016;**213**:2281-2291

[16] Ulhaq SJ, Soraya GV. Interleukin-6 as a potential biomarker of COVID-19 progression. Médecine et Maladies Infectieuses. 2020;**50**(4):382-383

[17] Saji R, Nishii M, Sakai K, Miyakawa K, Yamaoka Y, Ban T, et al. Combining IL-6 and SARS-CoV-2 RNAaemia-based risk stratification for fatal outcomes of COVID-19. PLoS One. 2021;**16**(8):e0256022

[18] Sabaka P, Koščálová A, Straka I, et al. Role of interleukin 6 as a predictive factor for a severe course of Covid-19: Retrospective data analysis of patients from a long-term care facility during Covid-19 outbreak. BMC Infectious Diseases. 2021;**21**:308

[19] Liu F, Li L, Xu M, Wu J, Luo D, Zhu Y, et al. Prognostic value of interleukin-6, C-reactive protein, and procalcitonin in patients with COVID-19. Journal of Clinical Virology. 2020;**127**:104370

[20] Rose-John S, Winthrop K, Calabrese L. The role of IL-6 in host defence against infections: Immunobiology and clinical implications. Nature Reviews Rheumatology. 2017;**13**:399-409

[21] Cox MA, Kahan SM, Zajac AJ. Anti-viral CD8 T cells and the cytokines that they love. Virology. 2013;**435**:157-169

[22] Evans SS, Repasky EA, Fisher DT. Fever and the thermal regulation of immunity: The immune system feels the heat. Nature Reviews. Immunology. 2015;**15**:335-349

[23] Hou W, Kang HS, Kim BS. Th17 cells enhance viral persistence and inhibit T cell cytotoxicity in a model of chronic virus infection. The Journal of Experimental Medicine. 2009;**206**:313-328

[24] Hagau N et al. Clinical aspects and cytokine response in severe H1N1 influenza a virus infection. Critical Care. 2010;**14**:R203

[25] Dienz O, Rincon M. The effects of IL-6 on CD4 T cell responses. Clinical Immunology. 2009;**130**:27-33

[26] Kaiser L, Fritz RS, Straus SE, Gubareva L, Hayden FG. Symptom pathogenesis during acute influenza: Interleukin-6 and other cytokine responses. Journal of Medical Virology. 2001;**64**:262-268

[27] The REMAP-CAP Investigators. Interleukin-6 receptor antagonists in critically ill patients with Covid-19. The New England Journal of Medicine. 2021;**384**:1491-1502

[28] Rosas IO, Bräu N, Waters M, et al. Tocilizumab in hospitalized patients with severe Covid-19 pneumonia. The New England Journal of Medicine. 2021;**384**:1503-1516

[29] The WHO Rapid Evidence Appraisal for COVID-19 Therapies (REACT) Working Group. Association between administration of IL-6 antagonists and mortality among patients hospitalized with COVID-19: A meta-analysis. Journal of the American Medical Association. 2021

[30] Matthay MA, Luetkemeyer AF. IL-6 receptor antagonist therapy for patients hospitalized for COVID-19: Who, when, and how? Journal of the American Medical Association. 2021;**326**(6):483-485. DOI: 10.1001/jama.2021.11121